YOGA FOR A
HEALTHY MENSTRUAL CYCLE

Yoga for a Healthy Menstrual Cycle

LINDA SPARROWE

WITH YOGA SEQUENCES BY
PATRICIA WALDEN

FOREWORD BY
Alice Domar, Ph.D.
Harvard Medical School

 Shambhala Boston & London 2004

Shambhala Publications, Inc.
Horticultural Hall
300 Massachusetts Avenue
Boston, Massachusetts 02115
www.shambhala.com

9 8 7 6 5 4 3 2 1

First Shambhala Edition

Printed in the United States of America

♾ This edition is printed on acid-free paper that meets the American National Standards Institute Z39.48 Standard.

Distributed in the United States by Random House, Inc., and in Canada by Random House of Canada Ltd

Interior design and composition: Greta D. Sibley & Associates

Library of Congress Cataloging-in-Publication Data
Sparrowe, Linda.
Yoga for a healthy menstrual cycle/Linda Sparrowe with yoga
sequences by Patricia Walden—1st Shambhala ed.
p.   cm.
Includes index.
ISBN 1-59030-118-8 (pbk.: alk. paper)
1. Yoga. 2. Menstrual cycle—Popular works. 3. Menstruation
disorders—Popular works. 4. Women—Health and hygiene—
Popular works.
I. Walden, Patricia. II. Title.
RA781.7 .S6455 2004
613.7'046—dc22
2003025261

Contents

Foreword

A NUMBER OF YEARS AGO, A PATIENT FROM ONE OF MY MIND-BODY groups called me after the fourth session and said that relaxation techniques were just not working for her. I teach a different relaxation technique each week so by that point she had learned meditation, body scan relaxation, imagery, and breath focus. She had come into the group with multiple physical and psychological symptoms and she was miserable. She was isolating herself socially and struggling to keep up with her work. She reported that each time she sat down to do a relaxation exercise, it felt like a burden. Her mind wandered the whole time and she dreaded each session. She was sure that she was going to be the first patient of my career to flunk relaxation. I told her that the program still had six more sessions, which meant that she would be learning six more relaxation techniques. I was optimistic that at least one of these methods would provide some relief for her. As it turned out, the next session included a 90-minute introduction to yoga. I was unsure how she was going to do since she was in a fair amount of physical discomfort. However, about five days after the yoga session she called me and reported feeling absolutely ecstatic. She loved the yoga; it was the first time in years that she felt connected to her body, and she actually was achieving some peace of mind during her yoga practice. She went on to practice yoga on a daily basis and found that both her physical and psychological symptoms decreased.

All of the women who attend any of my mind-body group programs or weekend retreats are introduced to yoga. It is important for several reasons. First of all, the patients I see tend to be uncomfortable or angry with their bodies. They are either suffering from infertility, PMS, abdominal pain, menopausal symptoms, or breast or gynecological cancer. They feel that their bodies have let them down and are only a source of misery. Yoga uses the mind-body connection in a healthy way. It allows my patients to become more in touch with their bodies and to see that their bodies can lead them to relaxation and fitness. The gentle movements and poses they learn help them to use their bodies to their benefit and, for many of my patients, this is an enormous revelation.

The second reason why yoga is so important in my practice is that most of my patients are experiencing a chronic condition for which there may be no definitive medical cure. These women seek and receive help from the best physicians and nurses. However, many of the most up-to-date treatments do not provide complete relief for conditions such as PMS, endometriosis, or infertility. In cases such as these, it makes sense to avail oneself of the best that our medical system has to offer, and to complement that approach with techniques that can help in other ways. Yoga is easy to learn, it's free, it has no side effects (apart from an initial bit of muscle stiffness in those of us who are not in tip-top shape!), and can lead to wonderful physical and psychological improvements.

Think of this book as a guide—it can lead you to improved physical health, enhanced psychological health, and a wonderful sense that you are connected to your body in a good way. Enjoy.

Alice Domar, Ph.D.
Harvard Medical School

YOGA FOR A
HEALTHY MENSTRUAL CYCLE

Chapter 1
The Menstrual Metaphor

NO MATTER HOW OLD YOU ARE, YOU PROBABLY REMEMBER THE DAY you started your period. Perhaps you were in English class, in the middle of playing soccer, or out with friends. If you were lucky, you have fond memories of being cared for and honored by the important women in your life when they heard the news. But most of us have not-so-fond memories that include feelings of embarrassment and annoyance, coupled with plenty of physical (and emotional) discomfort.

Some things haven't changed much over the years. Well-intentioned relatives still warn young girls that getting their period means only one thing: they can get pregnant if they fool around. Siblings (and parents) still complain about premenstrual mood swings, and many a school nurse still lacks sympathy for a girl with cramps who just wants to go home.

Going through puberty is a hard journey. Having no support makes it even more difficult to embrace a monthly event that wreaks havoc on the emotions and makes your face break out, your body retain water, and your stomach hurt. Of course, the bad news is those symptoms don't miraculously subside when you turn twenty, thirty, or even forty. The good news? If you can learn to accept—and maybe even celebrate— these monthly changes, you can learn to embrace fully what it means to be female.

Menstruation is more than discomfort and bad timing. This monthly cycle embodies the essence of womanhood and as such plays a major role in every woman's search for mind-body wholeness. Yoga can help you discover this for yourself. By helping you tune in to your body, yoga teaches you how your cycle can be a barometer for your health and at the same time, connect you to other women you know—even to the earth. But before going for complete global awareness, you can use yoga and simple breathing techniques called *pranayama* to gain practical relief from cramps, heavy bleeding, and raging premenstrual syndrome (PMS).

YOUR BODY AS UNIVERSE

Have you ever noticed that you get your period at the same time as your roommate or as other women you spend a lot of time with? That happens a lot, and teachers of yoga and *ayurveda* (the traditional medical system of India) don't find it coincidental. In fact, they believe that

YOUR REPRODUCTIVE ORGANS

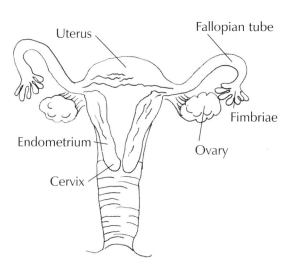

women's reproductive cycles not only mirror each other, but mimic nature, as in the lunar cycle. Every month the moon grows to fullness and then retreats into darkness. Your cycle works much the same way. Through a complex hormonal dance, your body prepares your womb to receive a fertilized egg. You move into fullness when you ovulate. Ovulation marks the time of month when you feel the most alive, bright, and full of energy; after all, as a human animal, this is when you are most interested in attracting a mate. Once a fertilized egg implants itself in the uterine lining (or conversely, you don't get pregnant), your energy recedes and your focus turns inward. The image of the dark side of the moon, like menstruation itself, is one of cocooning, reflection, and dreaming. You're directed outward when you ovulate (full-moon energy) and directed inward when you menstruate (new-moon reflection).

For some women, that in-between time so often characterized by conflicting emotions is the hardest to deal with. Annie, a third-year college student, didn't mind getting her period so much, but she struggled during her premenstrual stage. She said she often felt that her body needed to mourn the "loss" of the child that hadn't materialized that month, even when she had no reason to believe she was (and had no desire to be) pregnant. Her abdomen would feel bloated and crampy, her breasts sore and swollen, and her energy level drained—all symptoms of pregnancy. She often felt irritated or annoyed when her period finally came, almost as though she resented bleeding again. It wasn't until she understood more about the female reproductive system that she began to see how her emotions could play such an important role in her physical health.

Chapter 2

It's All in Your Head: The Physiology of a Healthy Cycle

CONTRARY TO POPULAR BELIEF, YOUR PERIOD DOESN'T BEGIN IN your uterus. The process starts in the pineal body, hidden deep within your brain in the recesses behind your eyes. This tiny, teardrop-shaped gland responds to changes in light and darkness and produces the hormone melatonin, which helps you sleep at night. According to British herbalist Amanda McQuade Crawford, author of *Herbal Remedies for Women: Discovering Nature's Wonderful Secrets Just for Women*, this gland not only registers and responds to the amount of natural and artificial light you're exposed to on a daily basis, it also signals seasonal changes and alerts the hypothalamus to begin your menstrual cycle. The hypothalamus, also a very sensitive part of your endocrine system, sits close to the emotional center of your brain and can react adversely to emotional upheaval or physical illness. The hypothalamus registers your body's most basic needs, such as hunger, thirst, sexual desire, and body temperature. When you're healthy, the hypothalamus provides the pituitary gland with what it needs to produce important hormones for reproduction. When your health is compromised, however, the hypothalamus may send out erroneous or incomplete information to the pituitary gland, which causes it to manufacture either too many or too few female hormones. That, in turn, throws your body out of balance.

Think of hormones as messengers that excite or rouse your body to act (hormone comes from the Greek word *hormon*, "to stir up"). The hormones from the pituitary—follicle-stimulating hormone (FSH) and luteinizing hormone (LH)—stimulate the production of estrogen and progesterone, respectively, in the ovaries. This action begins on the first day of your cycle, the day your period starts. On day one, estrogen and progesterone are at their lowest levels. The pituitary gland responds by manufacturing FSH, which in turn stimulates the ovaries to increase production of estrogen. During this stage of your monthly cycle, which lasts roughly 9 to 12 days until just before ovulation, an egg matures within one of the ovaries. At the same time, the increased estrogen allows the lining of the uterus (the endometrium) to develop and thicken, creating a safe and nourishing home in which the egg can grow, should it become fertilized. The increase in estrogen levels also improves circulation to the vagina and lubricates the cervix as a way of inviting sperm to enter.

When estrogen reaches a high enough level, the pituitary gland releases a surge of luteinizing hormone (LH), which causes an egg to leave the ovary and ovulation to begin. At this time, according to Christiane Northrup, M.D., author of *Women's Bodies, Women's Wisdom,* your body gives off hormonal signals (called pheromones) to let potential mates know you are fertile and sexually alive. Yet many women find it difficult to tell when they are ovulating. If you pay attention, you'll probably notice a watery, whitish vaginal discharge on the twelfth day of your cycle; that "fertile flow" indicates that you are ovulating. It may be followed, about ten days later, by additional hormonal fluctuations—known to most women as premenstrual syndrome (PMS)—which tend to be at their worst around day 22 of your cycle. These fluctuations, or warning signs, which include bloating, swollen or tender breasts, cramps, moodiness, or fatigue, let you know that your period is about to begin. If you

YOUR ENDOCRINE AND REPRODUCTIVE SYSTEMS

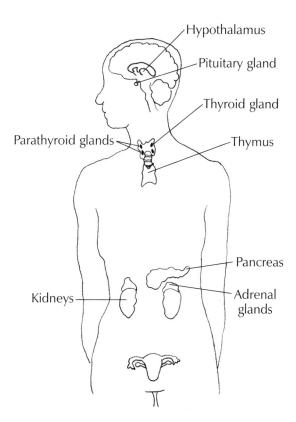

Hypothalamus

Pituitary gland

Thyroid gland

Parathyroid glands

Thymus

Pancreas

Kidneys

Adrenal glands

don't ovulate—and many women don't, especially when they first start to menstruate—it's almost impossible to tell when your period is due. It just shows up, and not necessarily on a schedule.

Once the egg leaves the ovary, your body prepares for a possible pregnancy. The hormone progesterone helps that happen. Manufactured by the corpus luteum, progesterone brings nourishment to the uterus

A Balancing Act

Estrogen plays an increasingly important role as your body blossoms in puberty. It shapes your secondary sex characteristics, giving you rounder breasts, pubic hair, a feminine voice, and broader hips. It also governs the first half of your menstrual cycle, which prepares you for ovulation and reproduction. Estrogen is at its peak during this time and affects your emotions (after all, it starts to flow at the insistence of the emotionally charged hypothalamus). If your estrogen output is balanced, your emotions and your body are ripe with possibilities—you feel sensual, outgoing, and creative. On the other hand, if your estrogen is not in balance, you may experience radical mood swings and debilitating menstrual cramps—even fibroid tumors and infertility.

Progesterone controls the second half of your cycle, nourishing the uterus and, if you become pregnant, the placenta. If progesterone production is balanced, you may feel more reflective, intuitive, and in touch with your dreams during this second stage. Too much progesterone, however, can cause you to feel depressed, lethargic, and sexually unattractive.

through increased blood flow and forms a thick mucus plug in the cervix to keep bacteria out. If no pregnancy occurs, production of estrogen and progesterone plummets and the uterine lining (the endometrium) dissolves and is shed as menstrual blood.

To complete this monthly purge, your liver and kidneys break down any excess estrogen and progesterone that remain into waste products, which are then eliminated from your body, along with environmental toxins, through your kidneys. Sometimes your liver may not be able to do this job as efficiently as it should, so these unneeded hormones can remain in your bloodstream. Your body then has more estrogen and progesterone than it can use, which can cause such problems as heavy or irregular periods, acne, fatigue, depression, or digestive disorders.

AN ALTERNATIVE EXPLANATION

For too many Western women, menstruating is rarely a cause for celebration. In fact, getting their period is a nuisance at best and a painful, debilitating experience at worst. But through yoga and its sister discipline, ayurvedic medicine (the traditional healing system of India), you can come to appreciate the wisdom of your reproductive system. Ayurvedic physicians believe that women have a distinct advantage over men by bleeding every month, an advantage that often translates into a longer lifespan. In the first place, your menstrual cycle helps you achieve balance between activity and rest, between outwardly directed energies and inwardly directed reflection. In the second place, ayurveda teaches that menstruation purifies the body every 25 to 35 days, gathering all the detritus and toxins (called *ama*) that have built up over the month and moving them out of the body along with the menstrual blood. This ama includes anything that hasn't been digested—food, emotions, stressors—and has stagnated in the body. It's helpful to think of ama as sticky, icky stuff that accumulates in your body when something is amiss. If you've taken care of yourself during the month preceding your menses, your body shouldn't contain much ama, and as a consequence, it should have a relatively easy time cleansing itself—everything should move through your body's channels unimpeded. However, if you've eaten lots of junk food, partied a little too hardy, or endured lots of emotional upset or stress all month long, your body will have to work much harder to push the ama through. As a result, you may see a change in the way you feel just before or during your period. Your PMS symptoms may worsen, and you could experience sharper cramps or even bleed more heavily.

Patricia Says

When you are menstruating, you need to modify your yoga practice a bit. The following guidelines can help:

- Concentrate on poses that do not obstruct the menstrual flow and do not cause fatigue. If you do standing forward extensions or forward bends, support your head and keep your abdomen relaxed. Go into the forward extension with a concave back to help create space in your abdomen. If you have low blood sugar or feel dizzy, do not do forward bends.

- Supported supine (reclining) poses will relax your muscles completely and calm your nerves to help relieve stress, strain, and irritation.

- Some twists are fine; Simple Seated Twist Pose (Bharadvajasana) is a good one. But don't do twists that compress your abdomen; these poses may cause undue pressure on your reproductive organs.

- Never do inversions when you are bleeding. That includes Headstand (Sirsasana), Shoulderstand (Sarvangasana), Plough Pose (Halasana), and Legs-Up-the-Wall Pose (Viparita Karani) with a bolster under your sacrum. According to ayurvedic physicians, going upside down during this time confuses your body and restricts the downward movement (apana vata) of blood. From a Western physiological perspective, inversions pull your uterus toward your head, which causes the broad ligaments to overstretch.

A SEQUENCE FOR HEALTHY MENSTRUATION

To get the most out of these menstrual sequences, focus on creating space between your rib cage and your abdomen. Relax your abdomen, pelvic region, and vaginal walls. Pay particular attention to your breathing. Direct your breath wherever you feel constriction. If your abdomen feels tight, breathe into it to soften and comfort it. If you feel constricted in your diaphragm or around your chest and heart, direct your breathing there. If you have cramps, breathe all the way down into your uterus. Directing your breath in this way brings an internal focus to your practice and allows you to relax deeply, resting your entire body. The Sequence for Healthy Menstruation is gentle, nourishing, and designed to make you feel completely cared for.

1. Reclining Bound Angle Pose (Supta Baddha Konasana)
2. Child's Pose (Adho Mukha Virasana)
3. Head-on-Knee Pose (Janu Sirsasana)
4. Three-Limb Intense Stretch (Triang Mukhaikapada Paschimottanasana)†
5. Seated Forward Bend (Paschimottanasana)†
6. Wide-Angle Seated Pose I (Upavistha Konasana I)
7. Wide-Angle Seated Pose with a Twist (Parsva Upavistha Konasana)
8. Wide-Angle Seated Pose II (Upavistha Konasana II)
9. Inverted Staff Pose (Viparita Dandasana)†
10. Bridge Pose (Setu Bandha Sarvangasana)
11. Corpse Pose (Savasana)

†CAUTION You may want to skip or modify these poses due to health limitations or ability. Please read the explanatory footnote beneath the descriptions before giving them a try.

1. RECLINING BOUND ANGLE POSE (Supta Baddha Konasana) Place a bolster vertically behind you and sit just in front of it with your knees bent and your sacrum touching the bolster's edge. Put a folded blanket on the other end of the bolster to prevent any strain on your neck. Place a strap behind your back, at your sacrum; draw it forward over your hips, across your shins, and under your feet (see below). Put the soles of your feet together and let your knees and thighs release to the sides. Cinch the strap securely under your feet. Lie back so your head is on the folded blanket and your torso rests comfortably on the bolster; your buttocks and legs are on the floor. (If you feel any discomfort in your lower back, add some height to your support with a folded blanket or two. If you feel any muscle tension in your legs, roll two blankets vertically and place one under the top of each thigh.) Remain in this pose for as long as you like, breathing deeply.

To come out, draw your knees together, slip the strap off, and slowly roll to one side. Use your hands to push yourself up to a seated position.

EFFECTS This pose can help relieve menstrual cramps, spasms, and heaviness in your uterus; take pressure off your pelvic area; and open your chest, clearing your mind and calming your nerves during times of stress.

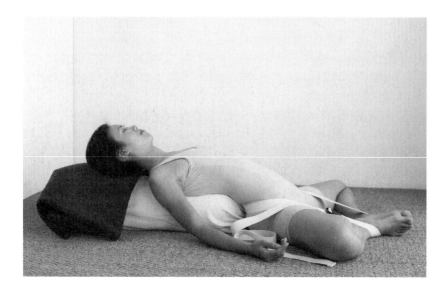

2. CHILD'S POSE (Adho Mukha Virasana) Kneel on the floor with two bolsters placed in a T shape directly in front of you, one end of the vertical bolster between your knees and the other end on top of the horizontal bolster. Spread your knees wide and straddle the bolster, bringing your toes together. Bend forward and stretch your arms and trunk up and over the bolster, pressing it into your abdomen. Rest your head on both bolsters and relax completely. Close your eyes, release your vaginal muscles, soften your abdominal muscles, and breathe into your pelvic region. Remain in this pose for several minutes, or as long as you like.

EFFECTS Many women find hugging the bolster into their abdomen relieves menstrual cramps and helps them release any tension in their muscles.

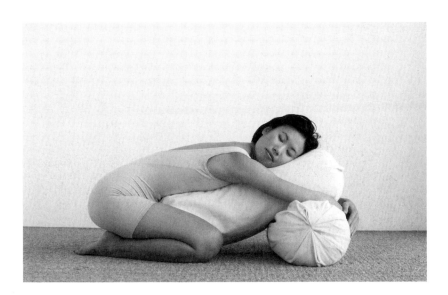

3. HEAD-ON-KNEE POSE† (**Janu Sirsasana**) Sit on the floor with your legs stretched out in front of you. Bend your right knee to the side and place your right foot against the inside of your left thigh. Keep your left leg straight.

Place a folded blanket or a bolster on your outstretched leg. Inhale, stretch your arms overhead, and turn your abdomen and chest so that they are in line with your left leg. Exhale, hold the sides of your foot and straighten your arms. Inhale as you lift from the base of your spine and move it in and up (your spine should be concave). Exhale, bend your arms to come forward as you lengthen your spine toward your foot. Fold your arms on your support, rest your head on your arms, and relax your abdomen and your brain. You should feel no strain on your neck, your back, or the backs of your legs. (If you do, sit up on a bolster or add more height to your support.)

Stay in this pose for 2 minutes, resting the base of your skull, your eyes, and your mind. To come out, hold your foot with both hands, straighten your arms and come up on an inhalation. Change sides.

EFFECTS This cooling pose has a toning effect on your reproductive organs and the supporting muscles. Many women find it beneficial for cramps, PMS irritability, or anxiety.

†CAUTION Do not do this pose if you are bleeding heavily, have diarrhea, or feel nauseated.

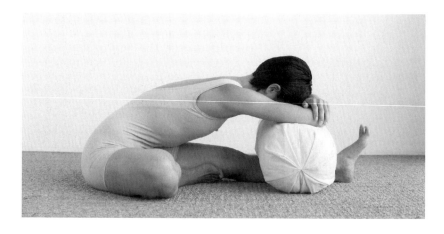

4. THREE-LIMB INTENSE STRETCH† **(Triang Mukhaikapada Paschimottanasana)**
Sit on one or two folded blankets with your legs stretched out in front of you.
Bend your right knee and bring your right foot back by the side of your right
hip, toes pointing back. Place a bolster or, if you're more flexible, folded blankets
on your left leg for support. Inhale, stretch your arms overhead and turn your
abdomen and chest so that they are in line with your left leg. As you exhale,
bend forward, reach your arms out in front of you, and lengthen your spine toward your foot. Inhale, clasp your hands around your outstretched foot or rest
your arms on your support. Exhale, turn your head to the side and rest completely. You should feel no pressure or strain on your neck, back, or the backs of
your legs. Breathe quietly in this pose for 1 to 2 minutes. To come out, hold your
foot with both hands, straighten your arms, and come up on an inhalation.

EFFECTS You may find this calming, cooling pose good for relieving stress, anxiety, and mild menstrual cramps.

†CAUTION Do not do this pose if you are bleeding heavily, have severe cramps,
or have diarrhea.

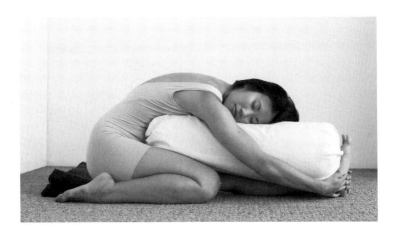

5. SEATED FORWARD BEND† **(Paschimottanasana)** Sit on your mat (or on one or two folded blankets) with your legs stretched out in front of you. Place a folded blanket or a bolster across your lower legs. Inhale and lift your arms overhead, stretching up through your spine and lifting your sternum and head. Keep your back slightly concave. As you exhale, hold the sides of your feet and straighten your arms. On an inhalation, lift from the base of your spine and move it in and up (your spine should be concave). As you exhale, bend forward and lengthen your spine toward your feet. Bend your arms and rest your head in your arms on your support. (If you feel strain in your back or in your legs sit up on a bolster or add more height to your support.) Press your buttocks into the floor (or blankets). Remain in this pose for as long as you like, preferably 3 to 5 minutes, keeping your abdomen soft. To come out, press down with your legs, hold your feet, straighten your arms, and come up.

EFFECTS This is a very restful pose that helps calm anxiety and relieve irritability, cramps, and headaches.

†CAUTION Do not do this pose if you have diarrhea or feel nauseated.

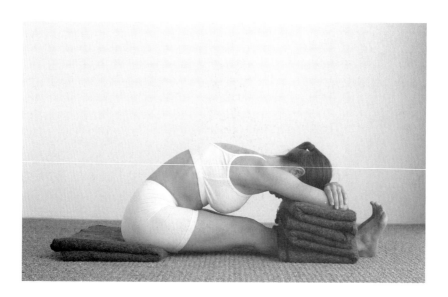

6. WIDE-ANGLE SEATED POSE I (Upavistha Konasana I) Sit against the wall and spread your legs wide apart; extend your ankles and spread and extend your toes. Adjust the flesh of your buttocks by drawing it behind you and out to the sides. If you find it hard to sit up straight in this position, sit on a bolster or the edge of two or more folded blankets positioned against the wall. This helps you sit up on your sitting bones. Place your hands on the floor behind you and, moving from the base of your spine, lift and expand your chest. Placing your hands on the floor behind you helps you lengthen up through your lower spine. Sit up tall and press down through your legs. Stay in the pose for 30 seconds to 1 minute. To come out, bend your knees and draw your legs together.

EFFECTS This pose can help the circulation in your pelvic area, regulate your menstrual flow, and stimulate your ovaries.

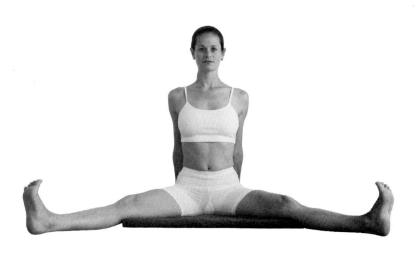

7. WIDE-ANGLE SEATED POSE WITH A TWIST (Parsva Upavistha Konasana) Sit up tall with your legs wide apart. Extend your ankles and lengthen your toes. Adjust the flesh of your buttocks by drawing it behind you and out to the sides. Place a bolster lengthwise on your right leg. Turn your abdomen, chest, and rib cage so you are facing your right leg. As you exhale, extend your trunk forward over your leg and fold your arms on the bolster to cradle your head. Your body should rest without effort; there should be no strain on your hamstrings, shoulders, or neck. Rest comfortably in this pose for 30 seconds to 2 minutes, relaxing your head, the base of your skull, your eyes, and your mind. Inhale as you come up, and change sides, placing the bolster on your left leg.

EFFECTS The gentle twisting action of this pose may help improve circulation in your pelvis, regulate your menstrual flow, and stimulate your ovaries and kidneys.

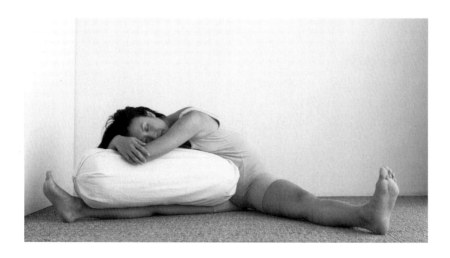

8. WIDE-ANGLE SEATED POSE II (Upavistha Konasana II)   Do Wide-Angle Seated Pose I as described above, but place a vertical bolster in front of you. Inhale and lift your arms over your head, stretching up through your spine and lifting your sternum and head. Keep your back slightly concave. As you exhale, bend forward, reach your arms out in front of you, and lengthen your spine toward your feet. Inhale, bend your arms, and as you exhale, rest your head in your arms on your support. Stay in this pose for 2 to 5 minutes. To come up, place your hands on either side of the bolster and sit up slowly. Release your legs.

EFFECTS   This pose can help blood circulate in your pelvis, regulate your menstrual flow, and calm agitation and irritability.

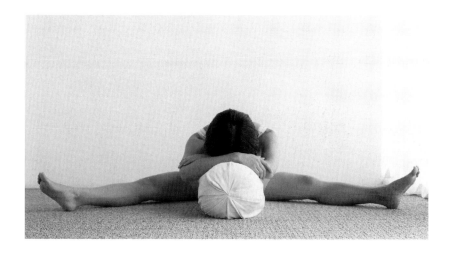

9. INVERTED STAFF POSE† **(Viparita Dandasana)** Place a folded blanket on a chair about 2 feet from the wall—far enough away so your feet can press into the wall when your legs are outstretched. Pile two bolsters against the wall for your feet, and put a bolster (and a folded blanket, if necessary) in front of the chair for your head. Sit facing the wall, with your feet through the chair back. Hold on to the sides of the chair and support yourself on your elbows, as you arch back slowly. Your head, neck, and shoulders should extend past the chair seat and your shoulder blades should touch the front edge of the seat.

Still holding the sides of the chair, arch back so your shoulder blades are at the front edge of the seat and your head can rest on its support. (You may need to scoot your buttocks farther toward the back of the seat.) Put your feet on top of the bolsters and against the wall, legs slightly bent, and hold the back legs or sides of the chair. Straighten your legs, pressing your feet into the wall, and roll your thighs in toward each other. Rest your head on the bolster. Keep your hands on the chair sides or legs. Breathe quietly for 30 to 60 seconds.

To come out, bend your knees and place your feet flat on the floor. Grasp the sides of the chair back and lift up from your sternum. Lean over the chair back for a few breaths to release your back.

EFFECTS This is an excellent pose when you're suffering from depression or fatigue. It opens your chest, which can improve respiration and circulation, help lift your spirits, and invigorate your whole body.

†CAUTION Do not do this pose if you have neck or back problems.

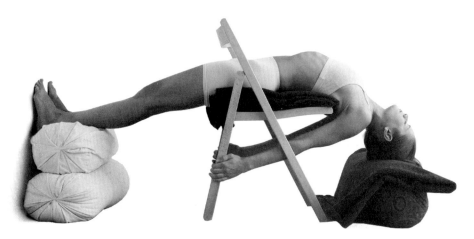

10. BRIDGE POSE (Setu Bandha Sarvangasana) Place one bolster horizontally against the wall and another vertically, forming a T shape. Sit on the end of the vertical bolster that is closest to the wall. Keeping your knees bent, lie back over the bolster. Slide down until the end of the bolster is in the middle of your back and your shoulders just reach the floor. Rest your shoulders and head on the floor. Stretch your legs toward the wall and put your heels on the horizontal bolster so your feet touch the wall. Your legs should be about hip-width apart with your feet pointing toward the ceiling. Close your eyes and relax completely, softening your abdomen and breathing deeply. Stay in this position for at least 3 to 5 minutes.

To come out, bend your knees and slowly roll to one side. Push up to a seated position.

EFFECTS This restful pose can be beneficial for depression, as well as anxiety and irritability.

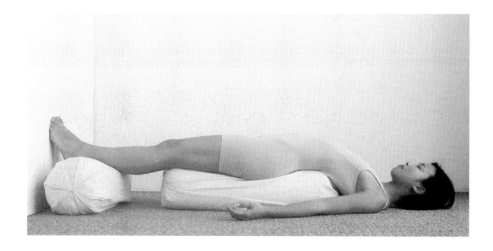

11. CORPSE POSE (Savasana) Lie on your back with your legs stretched out in front of you and your eyes closed completely. (Use a folded blanket to support your head, if necessary.) Place your arms comfortably at your sides, slightly away from your torso, with your palms facing upward. Actively stretch your arms and legs away from you and then allow them to release completely. With soft inhalations and quiet exhalations, surrender your body to the floor, without tensing your throat, neck, or diaphragm. Sense that your muscles are releasing from the bones and your skin is releasing from the muscles. Relax your eyes, ears, facial skin, and tongue and, as you exhale, feel your external organs resting against your back body. Keep your abdomen soft and relaxed, and release your lower back. Spread your awareness—your mind—through your body and let it come to rest in the heart. Remain in the pose, breathing normally, for 5 to 10 minutes. To come out, bend your knees, roll to one side, remain there for a few breaths, and then open your eyes and push yourself up with your hands.

EFFECTS This deeply relaxing pose allows you to release your abdominal muscles and vaginal walls. It helps relieve fatigue, as well as abdominal and lower back cramps.

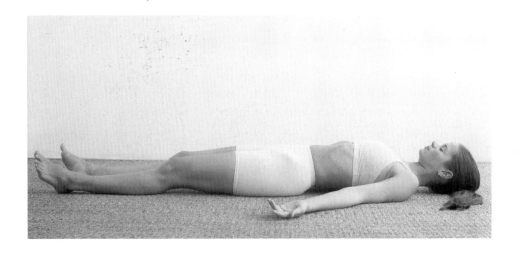

A SEQUENCE FOR JOINT ACHES DURING MENSTRUATION

According to Geeta Iyengar, B. K. S. Iyengar's daughter and an expert on women's health, if you have stiff or achy joints you can still work on those areas during menstruation without being aggressive. Take the time to slowly and gradually release and relieve your joints by doing the following sequence, which is particularly beneficial for women over forty. These poses help increase flexibility, lubricate your joints, and reduce any swelling or pain in your legs, knees, feet, shoulders, and hands.

1. Hero Pose (Virasana) Cycle
2. Reclining Hero Pose (Supta Virasana)

1. HERO POSE (Virasana) CYCLE Kneel on a folded blanket with your knees together and your feet pointing straight back, slightly wider than your hips. (If you feel any pressure in your knees, legs, or lower back, spread your knees farther apart.) Sit between your feet on a block or a bolster. You will move from this pose directly into the next, so place a bolster vertically behind you. You will not use the bolsters in this pose.

ARMS OVERHEAD (Parvatasana) Stretch your arms out in front of you with the palms facing you; interlock your fingers. Turn your palms away from you and stretch your arms overhead (A). Press your palms toward the ceiling and lengthen up through your inner arms. Move your shoulder blades into your back ribs, lift your sternum (breastbone), and stretch your trunk up from the bones in your buttocks. Hold this pose for 10 to 20 seconds. Sitting up tall and stretching from your waist, bring your arms down, reverse the interlock of your fingers, and repeat.

A

COW-FACE (Gomukhasana) ARMS Place your left forearm against your back, as far up as you can; the back of your hand is against your back. Reach your right arm over your head and, bending at the elbow, reach down your back toward your left hand. Interlace your fingers (or hold a strap if you can't catch your hands). Keep your right elbow pointing toward the ceiling and your head up (B). Roll your right shoulder back and bring your left armpit forward to open your chest. Be careful not to push your diaphragm and abdomen forward and keep your spine lengthening. Breathe normally in this pose for 30 seconds to a minute. Repeat with your arms reversed.

B

PRAYER (Namaste) HANDS Bring your palms together behind your back with your fingers pointing down toward your waist. Turn your hands so your fingers go in toward your waist and then up your back so they point toward the ceiling. Move your hands up the middle of your back, pressing your palms together. Roll your shoulders back while you spread and lift your chest. Push your elbows back (C). (If this is too difficult, fold your arms behind your back and cup an elbow in each hand to work on broadening your chest.) Hold this arm position for 60 seconds before releasing and stretching your arms to the side with your palms up. Do not shake your wrists; instead, stretch through your elbows, wrists, and fingers.

EFFECTS This pose is recommended to help ease swelling in your legs and prevent varicose veins. The different arm positions are excellent for keeping your chest open and your shoulders and upper back flexible. They also increase mobility in your wrist, finger, and elbow joints, as well as your neck.

C

2. RECLINING HERO POSE (Supta Virasana) From Hero Pose (Virasana), lean back onto your forearms and gently let your trunk rest on the bolster behind you, with your head on the bolster. Stretch your arms overhead and use your arms to lengthen your spine away from your buttocks and toward your head. Release your arms and rest them in a relaxed position at your sides. Close your eyes, and move your breath deep into your abdomen. Initially, stay in this pose for 1 or 2 minutes. If it's comfortable, you can increase your time to 5 minutes.

EFFECTS This pose stretches your hip flexors and is beneficial for the muscles and tendons around your ankles and knees. Because it is a gentle backbend, it will relieve stiffness in your shoulders and upper back.

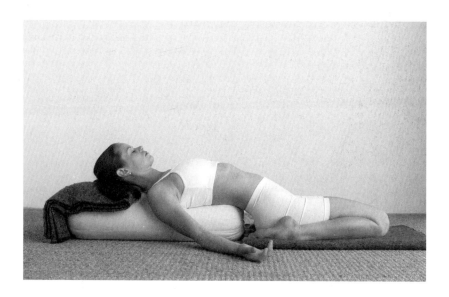

Chapter 3
Help with Common Complaints

SOMETIMES, NO MATTER HOW MUCH YOGA YOU DO OR HOW WELL you take care of yourself, you still experience problems with your cycle. Here are a few of the most common complaints women face.

AMENORRHEA

Amenorrhea is the technical term for not bleeding. Primary amenorrhea means never having a period. This becomes a "condition" only if a woman hasn't started menarche (her first period) by the time she has reached sixteen. Secondary amenorrhea occurs if you've had even one period and then, for any number of reasons, you stop menstruating. This is more common in the early teen years and in the years leading into menopause. It's actually quite normal for a young girl to begin her period without ovulating first. She'll have a light period one month and then no period at all for several months. This often occurs because the pituitary gland, which produces the follicle-stimulating hormone (FSH) and luteinizing hormone (LH) necessary for ovulation, is underdeveloped. As discussed in chapter 2, when everything is normal, estrogen builds up a thick, temporary lining in the uterus, which progesterone stabilizes following ovulation. If you don't ovulate, you can't produce progesterone. And if your body produces no progesterone, estrogen gets no signal to stop thickening the uterine lining. After a while, some of this lining begins to slough off and light bleeding will occur. Be patient. It may take a while for your body to establish its menstrual rhythm, but generally it does so without the need for medical assistance.

Unfortunately, many women panic too soon and allow their doctors to prescribe birth control pills as a way to regulate their periods. If they don't bleed regularly because they don't ovulate, birth control pills will only prolong the problem. These pills create anovulatory cycles; they don't correct them. They will, however, provide the progesterone the body needs to shed the endometrium lining that has built up. Most holistic physicians will opt to give a woman's body time to correct itself and prescribe gentle herbal tonics like chaste tree (*Vitex agnus castus*) to balance the glandular system.

Poor eating habits can also contribute to delayed menstruation. Women who suffer from anorexia nervosa don't have enough body fat for the menstrual process. Neither do female athletes who overtrain. You may think that's a blessing in disguise, because bleeding every month can be a hassle as well as physically and emotionally challenging. But if you don't menstruate, you don't produce the hormones necessary to build strong bones. These skeletal building blocks (estrogen and progesterone) ensure that you have enough bone density to lessen your chances of developing osteoporosis or osteoarthritis later.

Because the hypothalamus and pituitary glands are so closely connected to the emotional center of the brain, you may stop bleeding if you're under a lot of stress. Some women stop menstruating when their relationships fall apart; others find that a demanding work interrupts their regular cycles; still others are so frightened of getting pregnant that they don't have periods. Missing a period on occasion because of stress shouldn't cause undue alarm, but if it happens a lot, you should reevaluate your lifestyle, and you should certainly begin practicing yoga. Of course, recurring amenorrhea should be discussed with a physician, because suppressed menstruation can be caused by more severe medical conditions such as diabetes or thyroid malfunction, as well as extreme weight gain or loss or acute emotional distress.

A recent fad championed in women's lifestyle magazines encourages the continuous use of birth control pills to suppress menstruation completely. Having a hot date or taking an important exam on the first day of your period? No worries—simply take your birth control pills all month long and you won't menstruate at all. According to nurse practitioner Judith Obedzinski at Kaiser Permanente in Northern California, this practice isn't dangerous per se. By taking the pill, you're giving your body the estrogen and progesterone it needs to build peak bone mass. The only time she thinks this practice makes sense, however, is if you suffer horribly from premenstrual syndrome (PMS) or heavy bleeding and nothing has helped. Even then, it should be followed only for a limited time. But if you choose to go this route simply because of convenience, menstruation then becomes just a physical nuisance you want to avoid, instead of a powerful metaphor for being in the world and a tool for understanding who you truly are.

HOW YOGA CAN HELP

Yoga gets your period going in two very important ways. First, doing yoga consistently helps mitigate the stress that can cause your cycle to go off-kilter. Doing restful, restorative poses whenever you feel overwhelmed, overworked, and on edge will help calm your nervous system and give your reproductive system a chance to get back on track. Second, balancing your endocrine system may help the pituitary, thyroid, and hypothalamus perform correctly. Incorporate poses into your yoga practice (when you are not menstruating) that take your body through a full range of motion, paying particular attention to inversions, twists, and backbends. Patricia says inversions increase blood circulation and balance your endocrine system, backbends tone your liver, and twists massage your internal organs.

MENORRHAGIA

Menorrhagia means heavy bleeding. Just as you can go a month or more without a period, you can also have bouts of heavy bleeding. For the most part, such bleeding is normal, as long as the blood is bright red, you don't experience clotting or heavy cramps, and you aren't wiped out every time you get your period. When the bleeding becomes excessive—

Patricia Says

When you menstruate, and particularly during bouts of heavy bleeding, you'll want to change the focus of your practice.

- Don't try to get better or go deeper into a pose than usual.
- Never do inversions when you are bleeding. That includes Head-stand (Sirsasana), Shoulderstand (Sarvangasana), Plough Pose (Ha-lasana), and Legs-Up-the-Wall Pose (Viparita Karani) with a bolster under your sacrum. However, Legs-Up-the-Wall is a very restful and appropriate pose to do when you are menstruating, as long as your sacrum is not higher than your head.
- Relax completely into each pose. Soften your abdomen, let your brain relax deeply, and direct your breath to any areas that feel dis-comfort—your abdomen, your head, your back, and your legs.
- Don't do standing poses unless you do them against the wall. With the exception of Half-Moon Pose (Ardha Chandrasana), standing poses cause many women to tighten the muscles in their lower ab-domen and uterus. When you menstruate, you want your abdomen to be soft and your vaginal muscles to relax.

that is, when you continue to soak through several pads or tampons even on the second or third day of your period—something is wrong. In fact, if menorrhagia continues month after month, it can lead to anemia and iron deficiency, so see your doctor for an evaluation.

A variety of physical conditions can contribute to menorrhagia. En-dometriosis and fibroids can cause heavy bleeding. So can ovarian cysts. Not surprisingly, emotional upsets also cause the body to bleed excessively. Christiane Northrup, M.D., points out that chronic stress over what she terms "second chakra issues, including creativity, relationships, money, and control of others" may be the culprit for women experiencing men-orrhagia. She encourages her patients to set aside time to be creative, to mourn the loss of old relationships, and to learn to voice the joys and frustrations in new ones. When women heed the signals their bodies give them, she says, their periods often return to normal.

Marilyn is a good example of how emotions can influence the menstrual cycle. She left Southern California and settled in Chicago, where she supported her husband who was a university student there. She hated what she was doing, and she couldn't get used to the cold winters. As soon as the temperatures dipped below about 20 degrees, she would begin to bleed heavily, and it wouldn't let up until the thermostat rose above freezing and the sun came out—often weeks at a time. Several doctors examined her but could find nothing wrong. She kept telling them she thought her menorrhagia had something to do with the weather. They told her that was impossible. Finally, she sought help from an ayurvedic counselor. As Marilyn began to voice her unhappiness and her feelings of powerlessness, she felt more certain than ever that her body was trying to purge itself of all the emotional detritus she had been unwilling to face. Her body reflected her unhappiness and her inability to adjust to the changes she faced in a new environment; the warmth of the sun (to her, a symbol of returning home) brought balance to her reproductive system. Once she came to terms with her feelings and started to take action, her periods became more normal.

HOW YOGA CAN HELP

If you feel weak and exhausted from excessive bleeding, you can simply rest and not practice at all. Otherwise it's safe and helpful to practice the sequence for heavy periods that we've provided in this chapter. With the exception of Half-Moon Pose (Ardha Chandrasana), which is done against the wall for support, Patricia advises against doing standing poses. Standing poses require a lot of strength and energy; heavy bleeding zaps you of both. Half-Moon Pose, on the other hand, opens your pelvic region and brings space to your abdomen. Take care not to stay in this pose too long; instead, go in and out of it a few times. Overall, Geeta recommends choosing poses that conserve your energy or calm your endocrine system. Some favorites of hers and Patricia's include supine poses such as Reclining Bound Angle Pose (Supta Baddha Konasana), Bridge Pose (Seta Bandha Sarvangasana), and Reclining Big Toe Pose II (Supta Padangusthasana II), all of which use blankets, bolsters, and straps to support you. These reclining poses help relax your lower torso, slow down the constantly throbbing sensation in your abdomen, and bring deep relaxation.

In addition to the more backbending poses shown here, you may prefer to bend forward. In that case, simple forward extensions work well. Patricia recommends doing these poses fully supported so that your body doesn't have to work so hard to achieve benefits. You can't really relax if your hamstrings (the backs of your legs) are tight and sore or if you can't straighten your spine. Done restfully (with props), Child's Pose (Adho Mukha Virasana), Head-on-Knee Pose (Janu Sirsasana), Three-Limb Intense Stretch (Triang Mukhaikapada Paschimottanasana), and Wide-Angle Seated Pose with a Twist (Parsva Upavistha Konasana) all reduce bleeding, soothe your abdomen, and rest your head and brain. See the Sequence for Healthy Menstruation, beginning on page 11.

A SEQUENCE FOR HEAVY PERIODS

1. Bound Angle Pose (Baddha Konasana)
2. Wide-Angle Seated Pose I (Upavistha Konasana I)
3. Half-Moon Pose (Ardha Chandrasana)
4. Reclining Bound Angle Pose (Supta Baddha Konasana)
5. Bridge Pose (Setu Bandha Sarvangasana)
6. Corpse Pose (Savasana)

1. BOUND ANGLE POSE (Baddha Konasana) Sit against the wall with your back straight and your abdomen lifted. (If you have trouble sitting upright, sit on a bolster or the edge of two folded blankets so you don't round your lower back.) Bending your legs, open your knees out and bring the soles of your feet together. Hold the tops of your feet and draw your heels in toward your perineum (the pubic bone). The outer edges of your feet should remain on the floor. Lengthen your spine upward, leading with the crown of your head, and release your inner thighs from groin to knee. Stretch your arms out in front of you. Interlace your fingers, turn your palms away from you, and as you inhale, lift your arms up and overhead without tensing your groin. Stay in this position for 30 seconds or more, breathing normally. To come out, relax your arms and bring your knees up one at a time. Stretch your legs out in front of you.

EFFECTS This is a terrific pose to help alleviate cramps, heavy bleeding, and a feeling of heaviness in your abdomen.

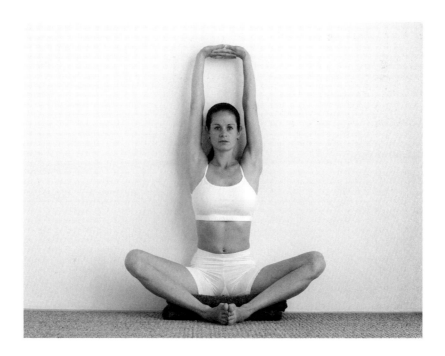

2. WIDE-ANGLE SEATED POSE I (Upavistha Konasana I) From Bound Angle Pose (Baddha Konasana), remain seated with your back against the wall, spread your legs wide apart, extend your ankles and spread and lengthen your toes. Adjust the flesh of your buttocks by drawing it behind you and out to the sides. Lift your arms over your head and clasp your hands together, palms facing the ceiling. Sit up tall, stretching from groin to heels and keep your knees straight. Stay in this position for at least 30 seconds, breathing normally. Take care to completely relax your pelvic area, vaginal walls, and abdominal muscles. To come out, lower your arms and draw your legs together.

EFFECTS This pose may be especially beneficial in slowing heavy bleeding associated with fibroid tumors and endometriosis. It massages your reproductive organs and gently lifts your uterus, which has a drying effect.

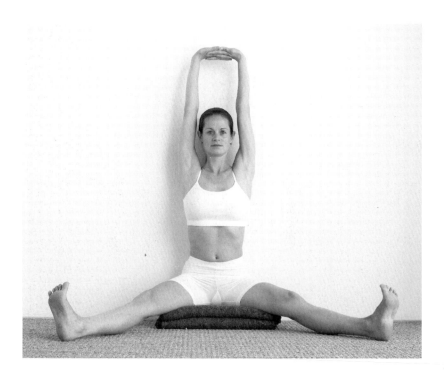

3. HALF-MOON POSE (Ardha Chandrasana) Begin in Triangle Pose (Utthita Trikonasana) (A): Stand up tall with your back close to the wall. Step your feet as far apart as possible, at least 3½ to 4 feet, and place a block near your left foot. Turn your left foot out 90 degrees and your right foot slightly inward. The heel of your left foot should line up with the arch of your right. Stretch your arms out to the sides, draw up through your quadriceps, and lift your abdomen and chest. On an exhalation, keeping your back straight, extend your trunk to the left and bring your left hand down to the block (A). Bend your left knee, pick up the block with the fingertips of your left hand and move it about a foot in front of your left leg against the wall. Come up onto the toes of your left foot. Exhale, simultaneously straightening your left leg and raising your right until it is parallel to the floor. Your right leg, hips, shoulders, and head should rest against the

A

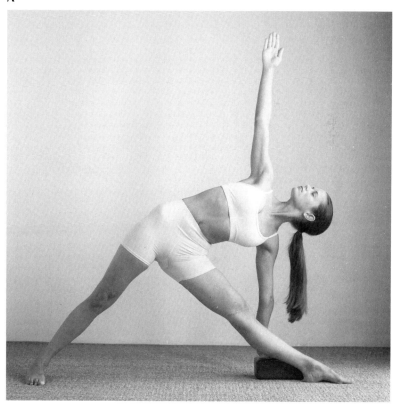

wall. Turn your pelvis and chest toward the ceiling. Stretch your right arm up in line with your shoulders and open your chest and pelvis further. Draw your shoulder blades into your back and look up at your right hand or straight ahead (B). Hold for 15 seconds, breathing normally.

To come out, bend your left leg, reach back through your right leg, and place your right foot on the floor, returning to Extended Triangle Pose. Inhale, come to standing, and repeat on the other side. End in a standing position with your feet together.

EFFECTS This is an excellent pose to help stop heavy bleeding and relieve the cramping associated with fibroid tumors and endometriosis.

B

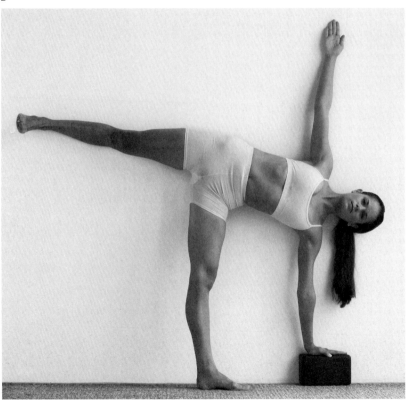

4. RECLINING BOUND ANGLE POSE (Supta Baddha Konasana) Sit in the middle of a vertical bolster with a folded blanket at the end of it for your head. Place a strap behind your back, at your sacrum; draw it forward over your hips, across your shins, and under your feet. Put the soles of your feet together and let your knees and thighs release to the sides. Cinch the strap securely under your feet. Lie back so your head and shoulders are off the bolster (and resting on the blanket) and your feet are on the bolster. Breathe normally, softening your belly and releasing your pelvic floor. Remain in this pose as long as you like—5 to 10 minutes at least.

To come out, draw your knees together, slip the strap off, and slowly roll to one side. Use your hands to push yourself up to a seated position.

EFFECTS This modified pose helps arrest heavy bleeding and relieves the heaviness in your uterus by taking pressure off your pelvic area.

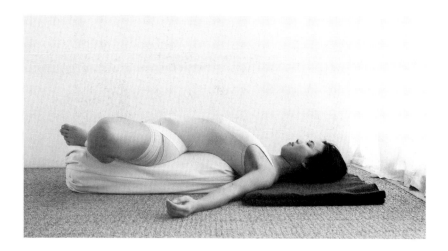

5. BRIDGE POSE (Setu Bandha Sarvangasana) Place one bolster horizontally against the wall and another vertically, forming a T shape. Sit on the end of the vertical bolster that is closest to the wall. Keeping your knees bent, lie back over the bolster. Slide down until the end of the bolster is in the middle of your back and your shoulders just reach the floor. Rest your shoulders and head on the floor. Stretch your legs toward the wall and put your heels on the horizontal bolster so your feet touch the wall. Your legs should be about hip-width apart with your feet pointing toward the ceiling. Close your eyes and relax completely, softening your abdomen and breathing deeply. Stay in this position for at least 3 to 5 minutes.

To come out, bend your knees and slowly roll to one side. Push up to a seated position.

EFFECTS Resting in this pose helps to relieve tension in your abdomen and heaviness in your uterus and acts to slow your menstrual flow. This pose is also good for melancholy or depression.

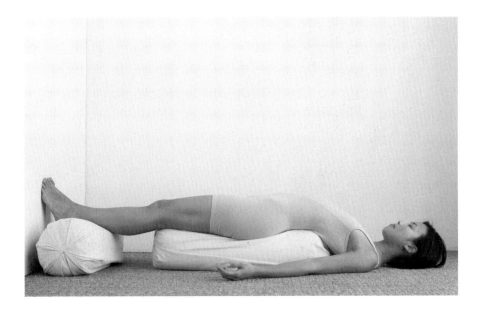

6. CORPSE POSE (Savasana) Lie on your back with your legs stretched out in front of you and your eyes closed completely. (Use a folded blanket to support your head, if necessary.) Place your arms comfortably at your sides, slightly away from your torso, with your palms facing upward. Actively stretch your arms and legs away from you and then allow them to release completely. With soft inhalations and quiet exhalations, surrender your body to the floor, without tensing your throat, neck, or diaphragm. Sense that your muscles are releasing from the bones and your skin is releasing from the muscles. Relax your eyes, ears, facial skin, and tongue and, as you exhale, feel your external organs resting against your back body. Keep your abdomen soft and relaxed, and release your lower back. Spread your awareness—your mind—through your body and let it come to rest in the heart. Remain in the pose, breathing normally, for 5 to 10 minutes. To come out, bend your knees, roll to one side, remain there for a few breaths, and then open your eyes and push yourself up with your hands.

EFFECTS This pose helps relax and restore your entire body and quiet your mind.

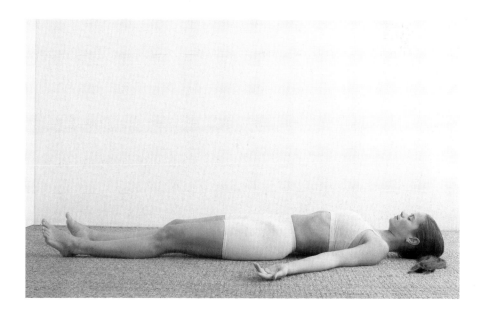

Chapter 4
Alleviating Menstrual Cramps

MENSTRUAL CRAMPS—THE BANE OF MANY A WOMAN'S MONTHLY cycle—vary widely in intensity and form. Some women, like twenty-four-year-old Sarah, get sharp, colicky cramps. Complete with constipation and periodic bouts of diarrhea, this type of cramp forces Sarah into a fetal position for the first twenty-four hours of her period. A friend of hers, who is in her early thirties, suffers from dull, achy cramps that lodge in her lower back and inner thighs and leave her feeling lethargic, bloated, and nauseated. Other women, no matter what age, complain of migraines, leg cramps, joint stiffness, and breast pain or tenderness that herald the start of their periods.

These women suffer from what is called *primary dysmenorrhea*, the most common form of menstrual cramping, which is unassociated with any other medical condition. *Secondary dysmenorrhea* is menstrual pain caused by something else going on in the body—pelvic inflammatory disease, endometriosis, or adenomyosis (a condition in which the glands in the lining of the uterus grow deeply into the uterine wall, causing the wall to bleed when you menstruate). Secondary dysmenorrhea can be quite serious, so consult your health practitioner if your cramps are un-usually severe, don't respond to dietary changes or stress management, or are accompanied by heavy bleeding. Although yoga can often help re-lieve the pain associated with secondary dysmenorrhea, the focus here will be on the primary kind.

Western physicians believe that primary dysmenorrhea is caused by an overabundance of the hormone prostaglandin $F_2\alpha$ in the menstrual blood. When this hormone is released into the bloodstream, it causes the smooth muscle of the uterus to spasm, which you experience as cramps. You can blame a diet high in animal protein and dairy products, as well as a lifestyle filled with unrelenting stress, for the presence of too much prostaglandin $F_2\alpha$ in your system.

Susan Lark, M.D., author of many self-help books for women, believes that primary dysmenorrhea occurs as either spasmodic or congestive cramps. Spasmodic cramps are most commonly found in teenagers and women in their early twenties. Women sometimes find this type of cramping subsides after their first pregnancy. Congestive cramps, on the other hand, make life miserable for women in their thirties and forties and seem to worsen after childbirth. Bloating, breast tenderness, weight gain, irritability, and headaches most often accompany these dull, achy cramps.

HOW YOGA CAN HELP

Any of the passive poses can help soothe cramps. Try several from the Sequence for Menstrual Cramps to determine which ones work best for you. Some women find relief in bending forward with something pressed hard against their belly. If that's your preference, try Child's Pose (Adho Mukha Virasana), while hugging a bolster or two. This pose, when done restfully, will soothe your abdomen and quiet your sympathetic nervous system. You may also find it helpful to do standing forward extensions, such as Standing Forward Bend (Uttanasana) and Wide-Angle Standing Forward Bend (Prasarita Padottanasana), as long as you rest your head on a chair or a bolster. Make the prop high enough so that you feel no strain in your hamstrings. Be sure to begin these poses with a concave back to ensure that your abdominals stay soft and you don't grip the muscles in your pelvis.

Other women prefer creating space in their abdomen. If that works for you, you may benefit from any of the supported reclining poses, like Bridge Pose (Setu Bandha Sarvangasana) or Reclining Big Toe Pose II

(Supta Padangusthasana II), which allow your breath to flow freely and release your abdominal muscles. These supine poses completely restore the nerves that have been under a great deal of strain and irritation. If you suffer from dull, achy cramps in your back, you may prefer a gentle twist, such as Wide-Angle Seated Pose with a Twist (Parsva Upavistha Konasana) with your whole body resting on a bolster. Experiment until you find something that relieves your type of pain.

No matter which poses you choose, don't worry about getting better or further along in your practice. Give up trying to get your leg straighter or your back more open, and focus on caring for yourself and purifying each cell of your body by bathing it in the breath. Bri Maya Tiwari, an ayurvedic healer, says that if you pamper yourself on the first full day of your period—no work, no worries, no cooking, no cleaning—your reproductive health will improve enormously. So do these poses as though you were treating yourself to an hour or so of pure indulgence.

A SEQUENCE FOR MENSTRUAL CRAMPS

1. Wide-Angle Seated Pose with a Twist (Parsva Upavistha Konasana)
2. Child's Pose (Adho Mukha Virasana)
3. Half-Moon Pose (Ardha Chandrasana)
4. Standing Forward Bend (Uttanasana)†
5. Wide-Angle Standing Forward Bend (Prasarita Padottanasana)†
6. Reclining Big Toe Pose II (Supta Padangusthasana II)
7. Bridge Pose (Setu Bandha Sarvangasana)

†CAUTION You may want to skip or modify these poses due to health limitations or ability. Please read the explanatory footnote beneath the descriptions before giving them a try.

1. WIDE-ANGLE SEATED POSE WITH A TWIST (Parsva Upavistha Konasana) Sit up tall with your legs wide apart. Extend your ankles and lengthen your toes. Adjust the flesh of your buttocks by drawing it behind you and out to the sides. Place a bolster lengthwise on your right leg. Turn your abdomen, chest, and rib cage so you are facing your right leg. As you exhale, extend your trunk forward over your leg and fold your arms on the bolster to cradle your head. Your body should rest without effort; there should be no strain on your hamstrings, shoulders, or neck. Rest comfortably in this pose for 30 seconds to 2 minutes, relaxing your head, the base of your skull, your eyes, and your mind. Inhale as you come up, and change sides, placing the bolster on your left leg.

EFFECTS The gentle twisting action of this pose may help improve circulation in your pelvis. As you exert gentle pressure on your abdomen from the twist and the weight of the bolster, you may find your cramps lessen in intensity.

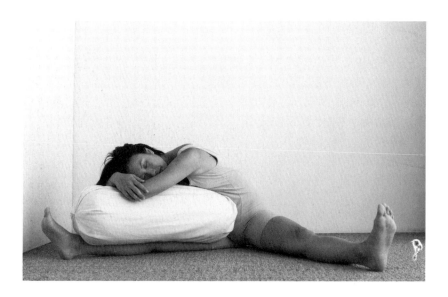

2. CHILD'S POSE (Adho Mukha Virasana) Kneel on the floor with two bolsters placed in a T shape directly in front of you, one end of the vertical bolster between your knees and the other end on top of the horizontal bolster. Spread your knees wide and straddle the bolster, bringing your toes together. Bend forward and stretch your arms and trunk up and over the bolster, pressing it into your abdomen. Rest your head on both bolsters and relax completely. Close your eyes, release your vaginal muscles, soften your abdominal muscles, and breathe into your pelvic region. Remain in this pose for several minutes, or as long as you like.

EFFECTS Many women find hugging the bolster into their abdomen relieves menstrual cramps and helps them release any tension in their muscles.

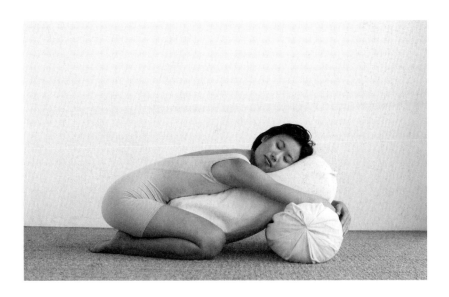

3. HALF-MOON POSE (Ardha Chandrasana) Stand up tall with your back close to the wall. Step your feet about 3½ feet apart and place a block near your left foot. Turn your left foot out 90 degrees and your right foot slightly inward. The heel of your left foot should line up with the arch of your right. Stretch your arms out to the sides, draw up through your quadriceps, and lift your abdomen and chest. On an exhalation, keeping your back straight, extend your trunk to the left and bring your left hand down to the block (A). Bend your left knee, pick up the block with the fingertips of your left hand and move it about a foot in front of your left leg against the wall. Come up onto the toes of your left foot. Exhale, simultaneously straightening your left leg and raising your right until it is parallel to the floor. Your right leg, hips, shoulders, and head should rest against the wall. Turn your pelvis and chest toward the ceiling. Stretch your

A

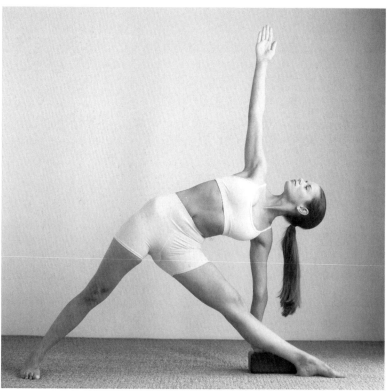

right arm up in line with your shoulders and open your chest and pelvis farther. Draw your shoulder blades into your back and look up at your right hand or straight ahead (B). Hold for 15 seconds, breathing normally.

To come out, bend your left leg, reach back through your right leg, and place your right foot on the floor, returning to Extended Triangle Pose. Inhale, come to standing, and repeat on the other side. End in a standing position with your feet together.

EFFECTS This pose is particularly advantageous for those who have backaches as well as abdominal cramps. The wall allows you to rest completely as you open up your abdomen and chest and bring more circulation to those areas. This pose also helps you relax your abdomen and vaginal muscles fully so you don't experience the tension and gripping that can make cramps worse.

B

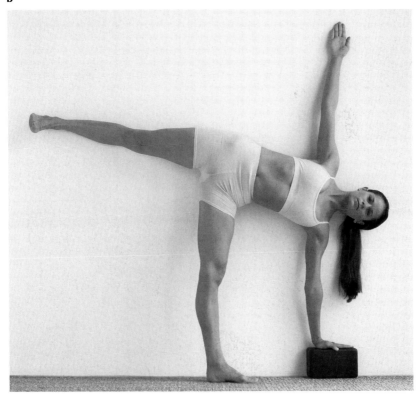

4. STANDING FORWARD BEND† **(Uttanasana)** Stand straight, feet hip-distance apart, with a chair cushioned with a folded blanket about 2 feet in front of you. Distribute your weight evenly between your feet and lengthen up through your inner thighs. Keep your legs and knees firm as you lift your arms overhead, stretching up through your waist and ribs. As you exhale, place your hands on the chair seat for support and bend forward from your hips, keeping your head up so that your back is slightly concave. Stay here for one or two breaths and then release your back and cradle your head in your arms and rest on your support. Breathe normally for at least a minute or two.

To come out, keep your legs active, put your hands on your hips, and slowly lift up to standing.

EFFECTS This pose lifts and tones your uterus and tones your liver, spleen, and kidneys. Supporting your head in this pose brings a sense of calm and peace when you feel agitated or anxious, which helps lessen the pain in your pelvic region.

†CAUTION Do not do this pose if you have body aches, low blood pressure, or low energy associated with a drop in blood sugar levels.

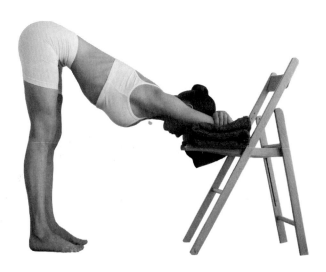

5. WIDE-ANGLE STANDING FORWARD BEND† **(Prasarita Padottanasana)** Stand straight with a bolster or two folded blankets placed about 2 feet in front of you. Step your feet apart about 4 feet (or as wide as possible), keeping the outer edges of your feet parallel to your mat. Tighten your quadriceps to draw your kneecaps up and keep your thighs well lifted. On an exhalation, bend forward from your hips, place your palms flat on the mat beneath your shoulders, and rest your head on your support. Keep your legs firm, but relax your shoulders and neck. Breathe deeply and let your trunk release downward. Stay in this pose for 1 to 2 minutes.

To come out, press into your heels, place your hands on your hips, raise your head and torso together, and stand up slowly. Step your feet together.

EFFECTS This pose allows you to soften your abdomen, stop gripping your vaginal muscles, and breathe into your abdomen. It also improves circulation in your pelvis and helps restore equilibrium to your central nervous system.

†CAUTION Do not do this pose if you have body aches, low blood pressure, or low energy associated with a drop in blood sugar levels.

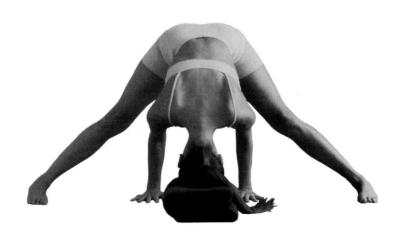

6. RECLINING BIG TOE POSE II (Supta Padangusthasana II) Place a bolster on the floor about 6 inches to your right so the bottom edge is in line with your right hip. Loop a strap around your right foot as shown in the photo, holding the long end with your left hand. Raise your leg straight up to the ceiling, run the long end of the strap behind your head, and straighten your left arm out to the side. On an exhalation, ease your right leg out to the side and down onto the bolster. Pull gently on the strap with your left hand to add a little resistance. Rest comfortably for at least 1 to 2 minutes. To come out, bend your right knee, release the strap, and hug your knee into your chest. Release your right leg to the floor and repeat this pose with your left leg.

EFFECTS This pose helps relieve lower back pain and ease cramps and general pelvic discomfort.

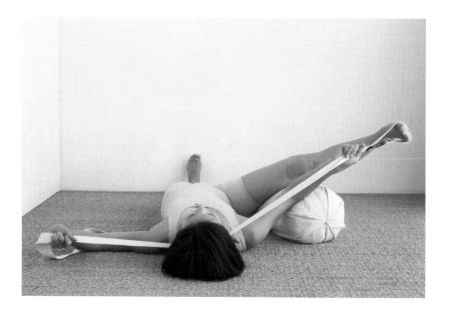

7. BRIDGE POSE (Setu Bandha Sarvangasana)   Place one bolster horizontally against the wall and another vertically, forming a T shape. Sit on the end of the vertical bolster that is closest to the wall. Keeping your knees bent, lie back over the bolster. Slide down until the end of the bolster is in the middle of your back and your shoulders just reach the floor. Rest your shoulders and head on the floor. Stretch your legs toward the wall and put your heels on the horizontal bolster so your feet touch the wall. Your legs should be about hip-width apart with your feet pointing toward the ceiling. Close your eyes and relax completely, softening your abdomen and breathing deeply. Stay in this position for at least 3 to 5 minutes.

To come out, bend your knees and slowly roll to one side. Push up to a seated position.

EFFECTS   Resting in this pose helps to relieve tension in your abdomen and heaviness in your uterus and acts to slow your menstrual flow.

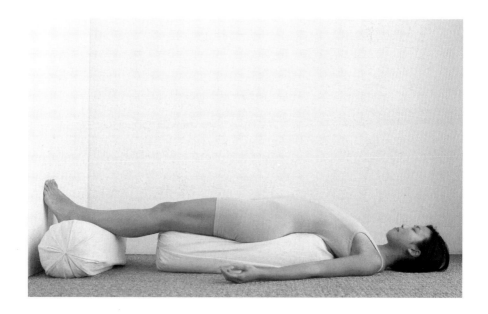

Chapter 5

PMS: Relieving Your Monthly Dysfunction Syndrome

A CATCH-ALL PHRASE IF THERE EVER WAS ONE, PREMENSTRUAL SYNDROME (PMS) can include any of more than 150 symptoms. Do you feel irritable, edgy, or "hot under the collar"? You have PMS. Anxious, moody, or light-headed, and barely able to remember your own name? You have PMS, too. How about bloated, achy, and depressed to the point that you could cry if someone looked at you sideways? You guessed it—PMS. You may also experience periodic bouts of acne, heart fibrillations, insomnia, herpes, hives, migraines, salt or sugar cravings, or even asthma, and these would all be PMS symptoms.

According to Christiane Northrup, M.D., the type of symptom doesn't matter much; it's the way it occurs. Generally speaking, she explains that women should see a pattern of flare-ups each month. Some women feel anxious and flighty about a week before their period, and as soon as they begin to bleed, they feel better. Others may get angry and rage uncontrollably two weeks before their period, only to fall into a depression the next week and feel appreciably better the first or second day of their period. Still others get intense sugar cravings—particularly of the chocolate variety—about ten days before they start. Giving in to that weakness may leave them with a horrific headache a few days later or achy, swollen joints until their periods start.

The jury's still out on what causes this common, monthly dysfunction that plagues so many women. Some findings, such as a 1998 study published in the *New England Journal of Medicine* (Jan. 22, 1998), suggest that PMS is caused not so much by hormonal imbalances, but by a woman's abnormal response to normal hormone levels. Other researchers contend that the emotional aspect of PMS cannot be overemphasized. That doesn't mean that the symptoms are "all in your head," as doctors even a decade ago may have led women to believe. But it does suggest that the severity of the symptoms may be directly related to the extent to which a woman's life is disrupted by stress and emotional upheaval.

By some counts upwards of 80 to 90 percent of all women (of reproductive age) experience some PMS symptoms, but not all of them suffer debilitating disruptions in their daily lives. Premenstrual discomfort, or PMD, is a mild form of PMS, characterized more by physical discomfort than emotional upheaval. If you have PMD, you probably have one or several of these symptoms: bloating, dizziness, headaches, cramping, joint pain, backaches, fatigue, constipation, or food cravings. You may find you can control these symptoms by monitoring what you eat, getting enough exercise (including a daily yoga practice), and relieving your stress levels.

PMS, on the other hand, which begins in the luteal phase of your cycle (usually 2 to 7 days before menstruation), clearly contains at least one or more emotional component. You may feel depressed or agitated, experience crying jags (for no apparent reason), feel fuzzy-headed or spacey, or overreact to events or people in a way you wouldn't normally. If these symptoms persist or worsen, you may have premenstrual dysphoric disorder (PMDD), a more severe disorder that can interfere with your ability to function—in your relationships, in your work, and in normal social situations. Symptoms include deep depression or despair, feelings of inexplicable sadness or guilt, inappropriate anger or hostility, confusion, withdrawal from social interactions, suicidal thoughts, nightmares, or fear of rejection.

PMS and PMDD can be difficult to treat, especially when no one is quite sure what causes these syndromes. One study out of University of North Carolina at Chapel Hill found evidence to suggest that women with PMDD had "more chronic stress in their lives on a daily basis" than other women. The study also suggested that women who have been sexually or physically abused during childhood are twice as likely to suffer from PMDD. The study, according to the findings posted on the university's website, found that these women's bodies responded to stress abnormally, with unusually high levels of norepinephrine (which increases heart rate, blood pressure, and blood sugar levels). Other possible causes of both PMS and PMDD include candidiasis, endometriosis, lupus, polycystic ovaries, irritable bowel syndrome, and thyroid imbalances. Some physicians prescribe selective serotonin reuptake inhibitors (SSRIs), especially if chronic depression predominates. Calcium/magnesium supplements often help, as well as yoga and meditation practices to decrease the stress levels.

Ayurvedic scholar and healer Robert Svoboda calls PMS a woman's "monthly dysfunction syndrome" and believes it to be a result of the disharmony created during the early part of the menstrual cycle. In other words, if you eat junk food, drink lots of caffeinated beverages, function with very little sleep, shelve your exercise routine, and consistently fail to deal with your feelings (especially negative ones like anger and hurt), you can count on problems later in the month.

Ayurvedic medicine postulates that a woman's biological rhythms are in tune with nature's own. Nancy Lonsdorf, coauthor of *A Woman's Best Medicine: Health, Happiness, and Long Life through Ayurveda,* explains that "anything that throws off our biological rhythms can create menstrual problems. Since each cycle operates in phase with every other cycle, if we are off-rhythm in our sleep cycle, this can easily throw off our menstrual cycle." Therefore, according to ayurveda, by regulating your daily routine, you can correct monthly imbalances and hopefully lessen PMS symptoms. For some women, however, PMS symptoms have gone on for so long they need herbal support, diet revisions, and major lifestyle changes to get back on track.

My favorite definition of PMS comes from Joan Borysenko, author of *A Woman's Book of Life: The Biology, Psychology, and Spirituality of the Feminine Life Cycle,* who calls PMS "emotional housecleaning," the time during your cycle that you have the opportunity to confront what's bothering you and release it. Suddenly something you've repressed all month long seems overwhelming and you just have to express it, get it out, deal with it. Women who stay in touch with their emotions and needs during this time often discover many of their physical PMS complaints subside along with their emotional components.

HOW YOGA CAN HELP

Yoga helps alleviate PMS in a number of ways. On a physical level, it relaxes your nervous system, balances your endocrine system, increases the flow of blood and oxygen to your reproductive organs, purifies your liver, and strengthens the muscles surrounding all these organs. Psychologically, yoga works to ease stress and promote relaxation so the hypothalamus can regulate your hormones more efficiently. It provides the time—and often the permission—you may need to go inside, listen to your body, and respond to what you hear.

The sequence on page 57 is designed to alleviate symptoms you already have. In order to decrease the frequency of PMS, however, it's important to practice yoga consistently. Done regularly, a well-rounded yoga routine should help. If you feel irritable or angry, do the poses with some form of support (see the PMS sequence) so you can rest your head

Patricia Says

- Soft instrumental music can help you turn inward, quiet your mind, and relax more deeply.

- Sometimes when you go to class during your period, you can get caught up in the energy of the class and end up working too hard. So, practice at home; that way you can gauge how much strength you have and can adjust your practice accordingly.

- Practice with awareness. Take care to work internally, not aggressively or muscularly during times of heavy bleeding, cramping, fatigue, or agitation.

on a bolster or chair. Resting your head cools your brain and eases any tension you may be experiencing.

Inverting—turning yourself upside down—is the best way to create balance and stability within your body's systems. If you feel irritable or anxious, Patricia recommends doing your inversions with support, as we've shown them in this chapter. You'll get the same results without having to work so hard. Headstand (Sirsasana) stimulates the pituitary gland and pineal body, both vital for good menstrual health, and increases circulation to your brain. For some women, however, Headstand can be too unsettling during PMS; they find that Shoulderstand (Sarvangasana) with full-body support gives them more freedom around the throat (thereby balancing the thyroid and parathyroid glands), opens the chest, and softens the abdomen. Plough Pose (Halasana) enlivens your adrenal glands and kidneys. This gentle inversion helps reduce swelling, especially in the legs, feet, and ankles; doing Half-Plough Pose (Ardha Halasana) may be easier if you suffer from lower back pain or abdominal bloating. If you feel depressed and lethargic, any of the chest- and shoulder-opening poses will help. For many women, creating this kind of space in the body quells the agitation they feel and lifts their spirits.

A SEQUENCE FOR PREMENSTRUAL SYNDROME

1. Reclining Bound Angle Pose (Supta Baddha Konasana)
2. Cross Bolsters Pose
3. Reclining Big Toe Pose II (Supta Padangusthasana II)
4. Downward-Facing Dog Pose (Adho Mukha Svanasana)
5. Standing Forward Bend (Uttanasana)†
6. Wide-Angle Standing Forward Bend (Prasarita Padottanasana)†
7. Headstand (Sirsasana)†
8. Shoulderstand (Sarvangasana)†
9. Half-Plough Pose (Ardha Halasana)†
10. Bridge Pose (Setu Bandha Sarvangasana)
11. Legs-Up-the-Wall Pose (Viparita Karani) and Cycle
12. Corpse Pose (Savasana)

†CAUTION You may want to skip or modify these poses due to health limitations or ability. Please read the explanatory footnote beneath the descriptions before giving them a try.

1. RECLINING BOUND ANGLE POSE (Supta Baddha Konasana) Place a bolster vertically behind you and sit just in front of it with your knees bent and your sacrum touching the bolster's edge. Put a folded blanket on the other end of the bolster to prevent any strain on your neck. Place a strap behind your back, at your sacrum; draw it forward over your hips, across your shins, and under your feet. Put the soles of your feet together and let your knees and thighs release to the sides. Cinch the strap securely under your feet. Lie back so your head is on the folded blanket and your torso rests comfortably on the bolster; your buttocks and legs are on the floor. (If you feel any discomfort in your lower back or inner thighs, add some height to your support with a folded blanket or two. If you feel any muscle tension in your legs, roll two blankets vertically and place one under the top of each thigh.) Take care to soften your abdomen and release your pelvic floor. Breathe calming breaths deep into your abdomen. As you exhale, let your abdomen broaden and recede toward your spine. Remain in this pose for at least 5 to 10 minutes.

To come out, draw your knees together, slip the strap off, and slowly roll to one side. Use your hands to push yourself up to a seated position.

EFFECTS This pose is excellent for helping you ease the anxiety, irritability, fatigue, and depression associated with premenstrual stress.

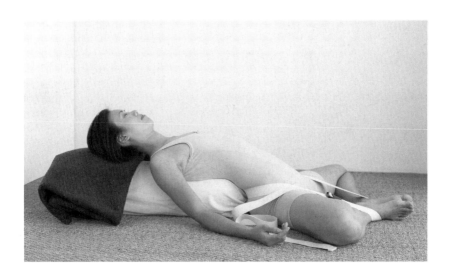

2. CROSS BOLSTERS POSE Place a bolster on your mat and lay another one across the center of the first to form a cross. Sit on the middle of the top bolster and carefully lie back so your spine is supported on the bolster and the back of your head touches the floor. (If that is too much of a stretch or puts strain on your neck, place a folded blanket underneath your head.) Place your arms on either side of your head, palms up, elbows bent, and relax completely. (If you feel any strain in your lower back, raise your feet on a block.) Relax in this pose for several minutes, softening your abdominal muscles and breathing deeply.

To come out of the pose, bend your knees and roll to one side. Help yourself up using your hands.

EFFECTS This pose opens your chest; improves respiration; and helps relieve the fatigue, headaches, and depression associated with PMS.

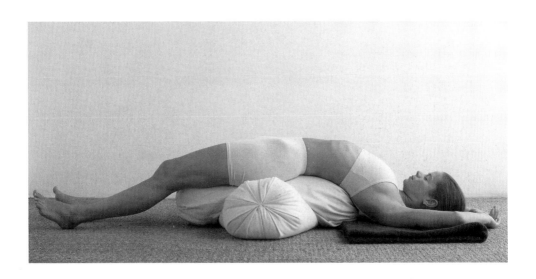

3. RECLINING BIG TOE POSE II (Supta Padangusthasana II) Place a bolster on the floor about 6 inches to your right so the bottom edge is in line with your right hip. Loop a strap around your right foot as shown in the photo, holding the long end with your left hand. Raise your leg straight up to the ceiling, run the long end of the strap behind your head, and straighten your left arm out to the side. Guiding the strap with your right hand, exhale as you ease your right leg out to the side and down onto the bolster. Pull back gently on the strap with your left hand to add a little resistance. Rest comfortably for at least 1 to 2 minutes. To come out, bend your right knee, release the strap, and hug your knee into your chest. Release your right leg to the floor and repeat this pose with your left leg.

EFFECTS This pose helps relieve lower back pain and ease cramps and general pelvic discomfort.

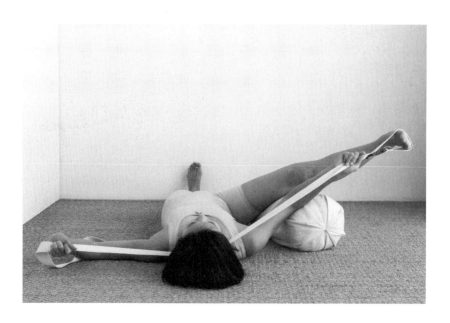

4. DOWNWARD-FACING DOG POSE (Adho Mukha Svanasana) To find the correct distance between your hands and feet for this savse, lie facedown on your sticky mat. Place your palms on the floor by each side of your chest with your fingers well spread and pointing straight ahead. Come up on your hands and knees, and turn your toes under. (If you feel agitated, have a headache, or experience fatigue with your PMS, place a folded blanket or two or a bolster vertically on the floor so it is in line with your sternum and will provide support for your head.)

Exhale, press your hands firmly into the mat and extend up through your inner arms. Exhale again as you raise your buttocks high in the air and move your thighs up and back. Keep stretching through your legs and bring your heels toward the floor. Keep your legs firm and your elbows straight as you lift your buttocks upward. The action of your arms and legs serves to elongate your spine and release your head. Hold this pose for 30 seconds to 1 minute, breathing deeply. To come out, return to your hands and knees and sit back on your heels.

EFFECTS This pose helps tone and relax your nervous system, relieving the anxiety, irritability, and depression associated with PMS.

Modification

5. STANDING FORWARD BEND† **(Uttanasana)** Stand straight, feet hip-distance apart, with a chair cushioned with a folded blanket about 2 feet in front of you. Distribute your weight evenly between your feet, lengthen through your inner thighs and roll your thighs in. Keep your legs and knees firm as you lift your arms overhead, stretching up through your waist and ribs. As you exhale, place your hands on the chair seat for support and bend forward from your hips, keeping your head up so that your back is slightly concave. Stay here for one or two breaths and then release your back and cradle your head in your arms and rest on your support. Breathe normally for at least a minute or two.

To come out, keep your legs active, put your hands on your hips, and slowly lift up to standing.

EFFECTS This pose lifts and tones your uterus and tones your liver, spleen, and kidneys. Supporting your head in this pose brings a sense of calm and peace when you feel agitated or anxious, which helps lessen the pain in your pelvic region.

†CAUTION Do not do this pose if you have body aches, low blood pressure, or low energy associated with a drop in blood sugar levels.

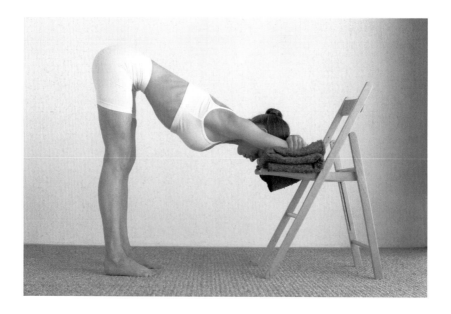

6. WIDE-ANGLE STANDING FORWARD BEND† (**Prasarita Padottanasana**) Stand straight with a bolster or two folded blankets placed about 2 feet in front of you. Step your feet apart about 4 feet (or as wide as possible), keeping the outer edges of your feet parallel to your mat. Tighten your quadriceps to draw your kneecaps up and keep your thighs well lifted. On an exhalation, bend forward from your hips, place your palms flat on the mat beneath your shoulders, and rest your head on your support. Keep your legs firm, but relax your shoulders and neck. Breathe deeply and let your trunk release downward. Stay in this pose for 1 to 2 minutes.

To come out, press into your heels, place your hands on your hips, raise your head and torso together, and stand up slowly. Step your feet together.

EFFECTS This pose allows you to soften your abdomen, stop gripping your vaginal muscles, and breathe into your abdomen. It also improves circulation in your pelvis and helps restore equilibrium to your central nervous system.

†CAUTION Do not do this pose if you have body aches, low blood pressure, or low energy associated with a drop in blood sugar levels.

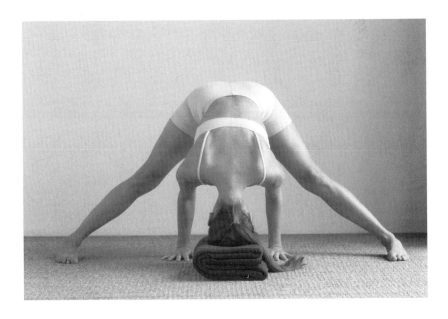

7. HEADSTAND† **(Sirsasana)** Place a folded blanket against the wall. Kneel in front of it with your feet and knees together. Interlace your fingers firmly, thumbs touching and hands cupped (A). Position your hands no more than 3 inches from the wall, your elbows shoulder-width apart. Your wrists, forearms, and elbows form the foundation for this pose.

Lengthen your neck and place the crown of your head on the blanket. The back of your head should be in contact with your hands. Press your forearms into the floor and lift your shoulders away from the floor. Maintain this action throughout the pose. Straighten your legs, raise your hips toward the ceiling, and walk your feet in until your spine is almost perpendicular to the floor. As you exhale, lift one leg at a time, and bring your feet to the wall (B).

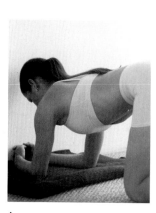

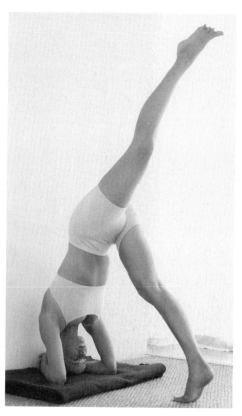

A   B

Keep your heels and buttocks against the wall. Roll your thighs in, lift your tailbone, lengthen up through your inner legs and inner heels, and keep your feet together (C). Remember to balance on the crown of your head, support yourself by pressing your forearms into the floor, and continue to lift your shoulders away from your ears. Keep your breathing even, your eyes and throat soft, and your abdomen relaxed. With regular practice, you can slowly learn to bring your buttocks and heels away from the wall. Hold the pose as long as you can, up to 5 minutes.

†CAUTION Before adding the next two poses, make sure you are able to stay in Headstand for 3 to 5 minutes with no discomfort.

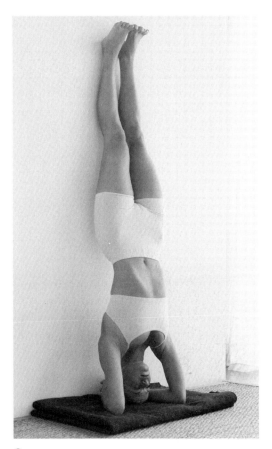

C

HEADSTAND WITH WIDE-ANGLE LEGS† **(Upavistha Konasana in Sirsasana)**
From Headstand, spread your legs wide, stretching from your groin through
your heels. Keeping your legs straight, stretch up through your spine and
broaden your chest. Remain this way for 10 to 15 seconds.

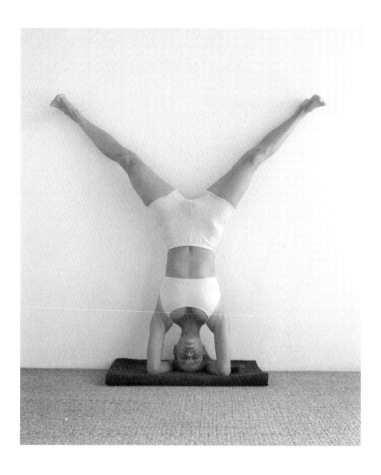

HEADSTAND WITH BOUND ANGLE LEGS† (Baddha Konasana in Sirsasana)
From the previous pose, bend your legs, spread your knees outward, and press the soles of your feet together firmly. Remain in this position for another 15 to 20 seconds, keeping your knees wide apart, and breathe normally. Straighten your legs and return to the wide-angle position, then to your original Headstand position.

To come out, exhale and bring your legs down to the floor one at a time. Bend your knees, sit back on your heels, and rest for a few breaths before raising your head.

EFFECTS This headstand sequence can calm the agitation and irritation brought on by hormonal fluctuations.

†CAUTION Do these poses only if they are already part of your yoga practice. Seek the advice of an experienced teacher if you have neck problems. Do not do these poses if you suffer from back problems or migraines.

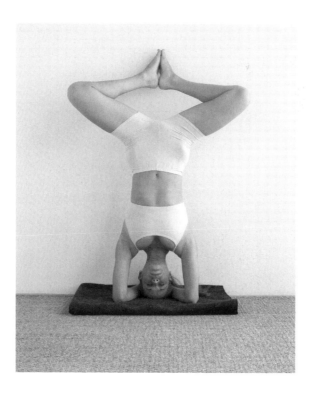

8. SHOULDERSTAND† (**Sarvangasana**) Place a chair about 8 to 10 inches away from the wall. Put a folded blanket on the chair seat, and two or three folded blankets in front of the chair. Sit backward on the chair with your legs bent over the top of the back; move your buttocks into the center of the chair seat (A).

Holding the sides and then the front legs of the chair, slowly lower your torso so your shoulders are on the blankets and your head is on the floor (B). Extend your spine and open your chest while doing this to get the proper position. Move your hands, one at a time, to hold the back legs of the chair; your arms should be between the front legs (C). Stretch your legs straight up, keeping your sacrum on the chair seat. Rotate your thighs in and extend from your groin to your heels. Close your eyes, bring your chest to your chin (D), and breathe normally for 3 to 5 minutes, or as long as you're comfortable.

†CAUTION Do not do this pose if you suffer from neck or shoulder problems, if you have diarrhea, or if you have a headache.

A

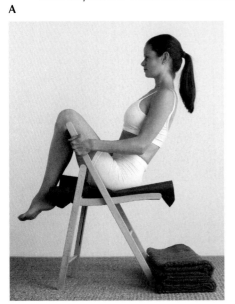

B

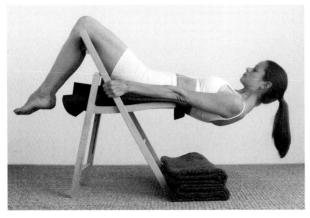

C

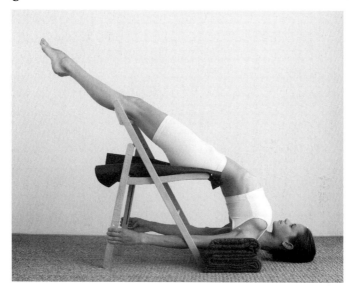

D

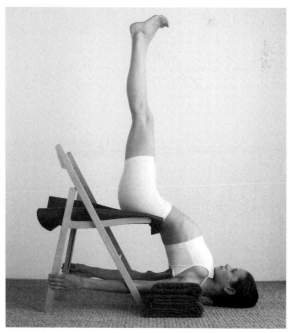

To come out, bend your knees and place your feet on the chair back (E). Release your hands, and slide down until your sacrum rests on the blankets and your calves are on the chair seat. Rest a moment, then roll to your side and sit up.

EFFECTS This pose provides many of the same benefits as Headstand. By supporting the head, this gentle inversion cools the brain and calms the nerves. Excellent for restoring energy.

E

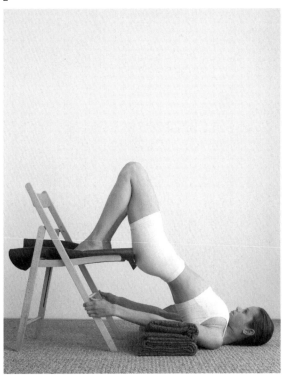

9. HALF-PLOUGH POSE† **(Ardha Halasana)** Place two folded blankets on top of your sticky mat with the rounded edges near the legs of a chair. Lie on your back with your legs outstretched, your neck and shoulders on the blanket, and your head beneath the chair seat. As you exhale, bend your knees and swing or lift your buttocks and legs, so your thighs rest completely on the chair seat. (Pad the seat with blankets if you need more height for your legs to be parallel to the floor.) Move your chest in toward your chin (not your chin toward your chest). Bend your elbows at right angles to your body and relax with your palms up and your eyes closed. Rest here for as long as you like—at least 3 to 5 minutes, if possible—breathing deeply to relax and quiet your mind.

To come out, place your hands on your back and slowly roll down, one vertebra at a time. Push the chair away, roll to one side, and sit up.

EFFECTS This pose balances your endocrine system and quiets your sympathetic nervous system so your mind feels uncluttered and your whole body can relax deeply. It helps relieve throat problems and congestion and may improve thyroid and parathyroid function. Resting in this pose lifts your spirits and helps tame irritability and anxiety. It is also excellent for premenstrual headaches.

†CAUTION Do not do this pose if you suffer from neck or shoulder problems.

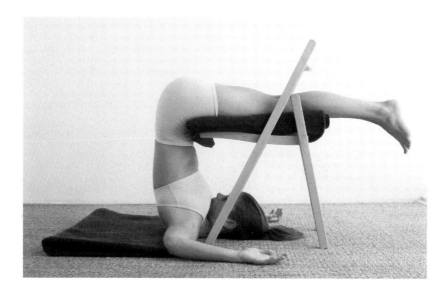

10. BRIDGE POSE (Setu Bandha Sarvangasana) Place a block vertically against the wall and have another at your side. Lie on your back with your arms at your sides and your knees bent. Raise your hips and chest as high as possible and support your back with your hands. Keeping your head and shoulders flat on the floor, lift your spine even farther, increasing the arch, and place the other vertical block under the fleshy part of your buttocks. Stretch out one leg at a time, resting each heel on the vertical block against the wall. Release your arms so that your hands reach just beyond the block under your sacrum. (If that's uncomfortable, bend your arms at right angles, fingers facing toward your head, and relax.) Hold the pose for at least 30 seconds, breathing normally.

To come out, bend your knees and place your feet on the floor. Then release the block under your sacrum and slowly roll down one vertebra at a time. Hug both knees to your chest and rest for several breaths.

EFFECTS This pose is good for toning and improving circulation to your kidneys and adrenal glands and for helping to regulate your menstrual cycle. If you feel irritable or anxious, try the supported version described on page 51.

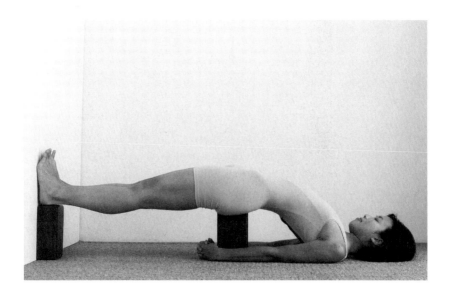

11. LEGS-UP-THE-WALL CYCLE (Viparita Karani) AND CYCLE   Place a bolster about 3 inches from the wall. (If you are tall, you may need a higher support, such as a folded blanket on top of the bolster.) Sit on the bolster so your right hip and side are touching the wall. Using your hands to support you, lean back and swivel your body around, taking your right leg and then your left leg up the wall. Keep your buttocks close to or against the wall. (If you feel stiffness or discomfort in your legs, push your buttocks slightly away from the wall.) Lie down so your lower back and ribs are supported by the bolster and your shoulders and head are on the floor (A). (If your neck is uncomfortable, put a rolled towel or blanket under it.) Extend through your legs and place your arms out at your sides, elbows bent and palms up. Rest in this position, eyes closed, for 5 minutes.

A

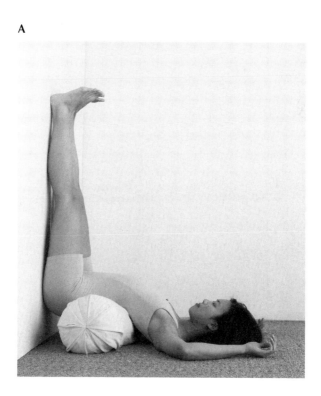

CYCLE Without moving your torso, allow your legs to open out to the sides (B). Remain in this position, breathing normally, for 3 to 5 minutes.

Again keeping your torso in the same position, bend your knees, cross your legs at the ankles, and continue in the pose for another 3 to 5 minutes (C).

Gently push away from the wall until your buttocks are just off the bolster and resting on the floor; the backs of your thighs and legs remain on the bolster (D). Rest in this position for 5 minutes, or as long as you like.

To come out of the pose, uncross your legs, rest the soles of your feet against the wall, and gently push away from the bolster, and roll to one side. Breathe quietly for a few breaths, then use your arms to help you to a seated position.

B

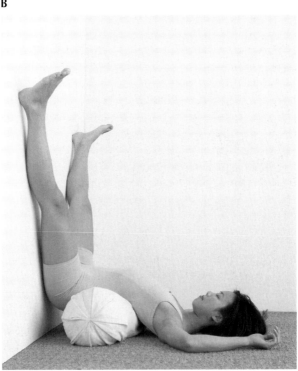

EFFECTS The poses in this cycle help calm your nerves, balance your endocrine system, relieve fatigue, and increase blood flow to your pelvic region. They also offer your body the complete relaxation it needs to heal.

C

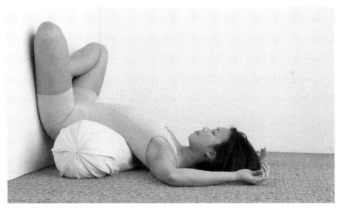

D

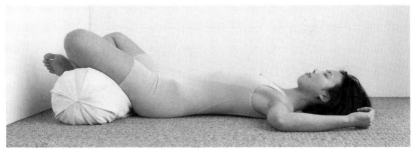

12. CORPSE POSE (Savasana) Place a vertical bolster behind you on your mat with a folded blanket at the far end of the bolster for your head. Sit with the end of the bolster touching your buttocks. Lower yourself onto the bolster and rest your head on the blanket. Relax your arms out to the sides, palms up, and let your feet relax away from each other. Focusing on your breathing, completely relax your shoulders, neck, and facial muscles. Keep your abdomen soft and relaxed and release your lower back. As you inhale, allow your breath to move into your chest, but keep your throat, neck, and diaphragm free of tension. Let your eyes rest and breathe normally for at least 5 to 10 minutes.

EFFECTS This wonderfully restorative pose helps relax your mind, quiet your nervous system, and rejuvenate your whole body.

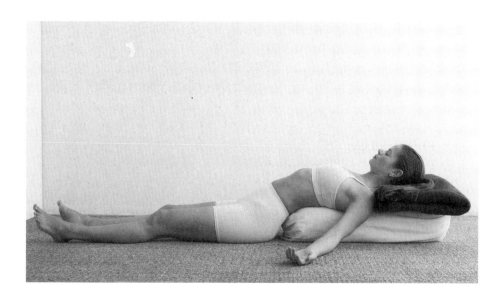

Chapter 6
The Physical and Emotional Causes of Endometriosis

SOMETIMES HEAVY BLEEDING CAN BE A SIGN OF A SERIOUS CONDITION, such as endometriosis, uterine fibroids, or ovarian cysts. Each can cause severe pain and result in an untimely hysterectomy. Under normal circumstances, the presence of estrogen during the first phase of the menstrual cycle allows the tissue that lines the uterine walls (the endometrium) to thicken prior to ovulation. With endometriosis, endometrium-like tissue shows up outside the uterus, most often on the pelvic organs, the side walls of the pelvis, the bowel, the ovaries (in the form of "chocolate" cysts), the fallopian tubes, the area between the vagina and the rectum, and sometimes the bladder. Endometrial growths can even appear on the lungs, thighs, and arms, or just about anywhere else in the body, except for the spleen. Cysts or lesions develop out of this wayward tissue and respond to the menstrual cycle in much the same way as tissue in the uterus—that is, it thickens as estrogen levels increase and it actually bleeds when menstruation begins. But unlike with uterine tissue, the body has no way of flushing out the endometrial renegades. Most physicians believe that's what produces the severe cramping, inflammation, and scar tissue associated with endometriosis. Because the body can't get rid of it, this misplaced endometrial tissue continues to grow, causing symptoms to worsen over time.

According to the Web site of the Endometriosis Association, endometriosis affects five and a half million women and girls in the United States and Canada and millions more worldwide. No one really knows what causes this often-painful condition. The most common theory, called "retrograde menstruation" or "transtubal migration," speculates that bits and pieces of the uterine lining break off and, instead of moving down and out of the body, move through the fallopian tubes and into the pelvis, where they attach themselves to the pelvic wall or the reproductive organs. According to Mary Schatz, M.D., a physician, yoga practitioner, and author of numerous articles on therapeutic yoga, a more reasonable theory posits that endometriosis occurs when cells in the pelvic lining mutate into cells like those in the uterine lining.

Some researchers believe that the circulatory system (blood and lymphatic fluids) carries endometrium-like cells from the uterus to other parts of the body. Others believe that endometriosis begins in utero (in an embryo) or that a grown woman's tissue has embryonic tissue memory and has retained the ability to create reproductive tissue out of nonuterine tissue. Still others hypothesize that certain families have a genetic predisposition for the condition. A very small study coauthored by Stanford University, the University of California at San Francisco, Vanderbilt University, and the University of North Carolina, Chapel Hill, and posted on the National Institutes of Health Web site, supports the theory that "having certain genes present in the incorrect amount contributes to the development of endometriosis." According to the findings on the NIH website, this genetic anomaly may also create "an inhospitable environment for an embryo to attach to the uterus . . . [adding] weight to the hypothesis that the endometrium of women with endometriosis is abnormal."

Research sponsored by the Endometriosis Association has pointed to environmental toxins as the likely cause of the prevalence of the disease. The organization looked at the effects of dioxin (a by-product of pesticide manufacturing, paper bleaching processes, and medical waste incineration) on the rhesus monkey population. Seventy-nine percent of monkeys exposed to dioxin contracted endometriosis. And the longer and more intense the exposure, the more severe the symptoms were.

Signs and Symptoms of Endometriosis

Having these symptoms doesn't necessarily mean you have endometriosis—you could have a pelvic inflammatory disease or another kind of infection. Check with your doctor if you experience any of the following symptoms for more than one menstrual cycle:

- Pelvic pain that worsens during or after intercourse or strenuous exercise

- Heavy bleeding during your period or spotting between periods

- Intense menstrual cramps, especially those that don't disappear after the first day of your period

- Rectal bleeding or painful bowel movements

- Inability to get pregnant

- Fatigue

- Leg or lower back pain

There's more bad news. Those who suffer from endometriosis are more likely than other women to have immune disorders, according to researchers at the National Institute of Child Health and Human Development. In analyzing feedback from a 1998 survey of 3,680 members of the Endometriosis Association, researchers found these women to be "a hundred times more likely to experience chronic fatigue syndrome than the general population," twice as likely to have fibromyalgia (pain in the joints, ligaments, tendons, and muscles), and seven times more likely to suffer from endocrine diseases. This population also had a significantly higher rate of allergies and asthma than women without endometriosis.

Whatever the cause, many holistic physicians believe stress aggravates endometriosis. Ayurvedic physicians recommend changes in diet and lifestyle, including lots of rest during the first day or so of your period, and gentle yoga asanas (poses) to relieve cramps, reduce stress, and deliver fresh blood to your pelvic region.

A number of physicians and healers agree with Christiane Northrup, M.D., who believes that endometriosis is a wake-up call for women who compete in high-stress jobs. She writes that it is often the way a woman's body demonstrates that her "innermost emotional needs are in direct conflict with what the world is demanding of her." In other words, if you consistently and relentlessly focus your energies outward and neglect your emotional and spiritual side, you may be a prime candidate for pelvic inflammatory diseases (PIDs).

CONVENTIONAL TREATMENTS

If a young girl suffers from endometriosis, her doctor is likely to adopt a wait-and-see stance, preferring not to order invasive procedures to correct the problem. Some young women opt to go on birth control pills in hopes that they will help—and sometimes they do. After all, birth control pills create anovulatory periods (periods with no ovulation). If you don't ovulate, you can't build up your uterine lining, so there is much less material to shed during your period.

If you are already well past puberty, your doctor may prescribe one of the new nasal spray medications, which are designed to block the gonadotropin hormone (the hormone that triggers ovulation). Or she may suggest that you take an androgen, a male hormone that chemically prevents the female hormones from producing your menstrual cycle.

There's no real way to tell whether you have endometriosis or another PID unless you undergo laparoscopic surgery (in which a fiberoptic instrument is inserted through a small incision in your abdomen). Nor can you readily tell how serious your condition is. Some women experience a lot of pain with very few endometrial lesions; others blessedly have little pain but more growths. Magnetic resonance imagery (MRI) or an ultrasound can identify other possible causes of your symptoms, but laparoscopy is needed if you want to be sure. Some women have had endometrial growths removed successfully (without relapse) through surgical means; for others, the growths and the pain soon return.

DIETARY SUGGESTIONS

Susan Lark, M.D., says high estrogen levels can "stimulate growth of endometrial implants." By concentrating on foods and supplements that will reduce estrogen, you may be able to successfully manage your endometriosis. Here are some of her suggestions:

- Eat more whole grains high in vitamins E and B complex, which can help reduce estrogen levels. In addition, the fiber in these grains will absorb excess estrogen and remove it from your body. Fiber also relieves constipation and helps rid your body of excess fat and cholesterol.

- Eat foods high in calcium and magnesium to ease cramps and muscle contractions. Eat plenty of potassium-rich fruits and vegetables. Potassium acts as a diuretic to prevent bloating. Beans and peas are excellent sources of all three of these minerals.

- Eat fruits and vegetables rich in vitamin C. According to Lark, vitamin C "facilitates the flow of nutrients into muscles and helps transport waste products out of the body." It also "strengthens capillaries, which helps reduce heavy menstrual bleeding." Eating more fruit will also help ease the cramping associated with endometriosis.

- Add soybeans to your diet. These legumes help lower estrogen levels and also provide plenty of bioflavonoids, which can reduce bleeding, especially for women who also have fibroids.

- Increase your intake of essential fatty acids. Adding a variety of seeds and nuts is a good way to do this.

- If you eat animal products, stick with fish because it contains essential fatty acids (as nuts and seeds do) as well as other minerals such as iodine and potassium.

Lark also suggests avoiding certain foods to help control symptoms:

- Red meat and poultry, which contain high amounts of estrogens.

- Dairy products, especially milk, cheese, and yogurt, which are loaded with saturated fats. These products contain arachidonic acid, which stimulates the production of prostaglandins. Although prostaglandins have vasoconstrictive and muscle-constricting properties, which contribute to the normal sloughing off of the endometrial lining during menstruation, excessive prostaglandin production in the endometrium can cause the pain, cramping, vomiting, and diarrhea associated with endometriosis and dysmenorrhea.

- Salt, which leads bloating and water retention.

- Sugar, which can cause muscle tension as well as depression and anxiety.

- Alcohol, which puts more stress on your liver and hampers its ability to metabolize hormones effectively.

THE AYURVEDIC APPROACH

Like many holistic practitioners, yogis and ayurvedic physicians believe that emotional and physical stress contribute to endometriosis. Remember the ayurvedic concept of ama, the sticky undigested experiences or foods left in your body (see chapter 2)? Ayurvedic physicians believe ama is responsible for preventing the downward movement of menstrual blood and forcing it upward instead. This retrograde menstruation causes endometrial cells to lodge elsewhere in the body. They explain that a woman has an aspect of life force, or prana, in her body called *apana vata*, which is responsible for the downward movement and elimination of all waste products. If apana vata is restricted in any way, the body cannot efficiently purge itself of menstrual blood, ama, and other detritus. Many women who suffer from endometriosis are also understandably plagued by constipation.

HOW YOGA CAN HELP

A consistent, supportive yoga practice can help you get in touch with—and remain aware of—your whole self, including your reproductive organs. Geeta Iyengar believes that "a woman's nature is related to her uterus." Therefore, she explains, "whenever [she] is exposed to any kind of physical, physiological, emotional, or psychological stress, she tends to hold [grip] the uterus." If a woman feels angry or tense, for example, she constricts her uterine muscles. So, according to Geeta and Patricia, when you are menstruating, stay away from poses that cause you to grip the uterine-rectal area, such as unsupported standing poses.

Practice poses that create an opening or spreading action in your lower abdomen. According to Geeta, this should bring you relief from the pain. Half-Moon Pose (Ardha Chandrasana) is one of Patricia's favorite poses for this. Sitting in Bound Angle Pose (Baddha Konasana) or Wide-Angle Seated Pose (Upavistha Konasana) opens and widens your pelvis. You can sit upright (against the wall if you feel tired) or lean backward and rest your head on a cushioned chair. It's most important to feel a lift in the lower abdominals above the pubic bone. If you can't feel that stretch or lift, prop your sitting bones (ischium) up on a bolster or a couple of folded blankets so you can.

Patricia says that if you suffer from endometriosis you should do asanas that facilitate apana vata. In other words, go upside down (since the apana vata is going in the wrong direction). Of course, you should never invert when you are bleeding. The inversions you choose should be done with open legs so you continue to feel the opening and spreading action in your pelvis. Do Headstand (Sirsasana) and Shoulderstand (Sarvangasana) with the soles of your feet together (Baddha Konasana) or with outstretched legs (Upavistha Konasana). If you do Plough Pose (Halasana), spread your legs wide as you lift them.

Once the pain has subsided, you can incorporate asana modifications into your daily practice that help heal any scar tissue that's left. You've worked to open the pelvic area and bring freshly oxygenated blood there; now you must knit things back together. Do your inversions and seated forward bends holding a block high up between your thighs.

Patricia Says

If you have endometriosis, avoid postures that tense or grip your throat or abdominal muscles, including arm balances. Don't do any breathing exercises (pranayama) sitting up when bleeding is heavy. Also, avoid performing any "locks" such as uddiyana or mula bandha. Otherwise you can resume your normal practice after you stop bleeding. The sequence in this chapter provides some important variations for you to incorporate into your daily routine that should help you manage your pain.

A SEQUENCE FOR ENDOMETRIOSIS

1. Staff Pose (Dandasana)
2. Bridge Pose (Setu Bandha Sarvangasana)
3. Headstand (Sirsasana)†
4. Legs-Up-the-Wall Pose (Viparita Karani) and Cycle†

†CAUTION Please read the explanatory footnote beneath the descriptions before giving these poses a try.

1. STAFF POSE (Dandasana) Sit on the floor in front of a chair padded with at least one bolster. Keep feet and legs together, hip-width apart, or slightly wider, depending on comfort. With your palms by your sides, press your thighs down into the floor and lift your spine up. Keep your legs active and extend through your inner heels. Look up toward the ceiling and gently lay your head to rest on the cushioned chair. The back of your head should rest comfortably on the chair with no strain to your neck or your back. If that's not the case, add more support to the chair (a folded blanket or two). Remain in this pose for at least a minute, if possible.

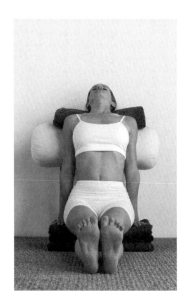

STAFF POSE WITH WIDE-ANGLE LEGS (Upavistha Konasana in Dandasana) Remain seated with your head on the chair and spread your legs as wide as is comfortable. Press your heels and thighs firmly into the floor and lift up through your waist and side body. Rest in this position for at least 1 minute or more.

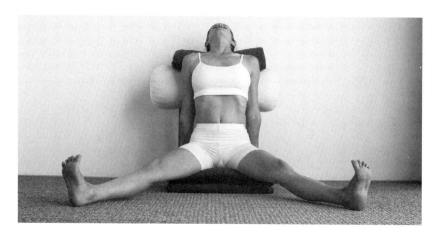

STAFF POSE WITH BOUND ANGLE LEGS (Baddha Konasana in Dandasana) Remain in Staff Pose with your head resting on the chair and bring the soles of your feet together (B). Rest in this position, with your hands pressing into the blankets, for at least 1 minute or more.

EFFECTS It's important to feel a lift in your pelvic region while you're doing these poses. The first pose creates a lift and stretch; the other two create an opening or spreading action in your lower abdominals to increase circulation to that area. These poses help alleviate the pain associated with endometriosis.

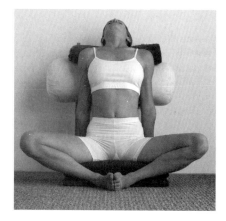

2. BRIDGE POSE (Setu Bandha Sarvangasana) Set two blocks vertically against the wall as shown. Place a bolster horizontally on the floor and a second one vertically across it to form a cross. Sit at the center of the cross and lie back so that your shoulders and head are off the bolsters. Stretch your legs wide, placing your heels on the blocks. Remain in this position for as long as you like, at least a minute or two. Use a folded blanket to support your head if you wish.

EFFECTS In this variation of Bridge Pose, you should feel a stretch and lift throughout your pelvis. Spreading your legs prevents you from gripping your uterine muscles and promotes complete relaxation of your pelvic floor. This pose also helps alleviate any pelvic pain you may experience with endometriosis.

Once the pain has subsided, and you are no longer bleeding, you can return to your normal practice. However, you should do the following variations of Headstand (Sirsasana) to help you heal any remaining scar tissue.

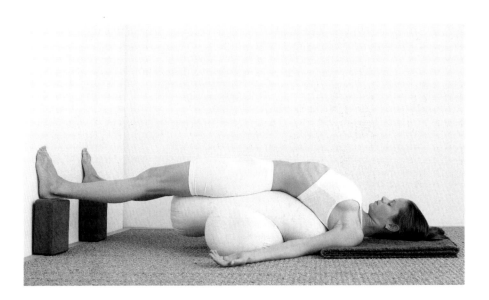

3. HEADSTAND† **(Sirsasana)** You may need an instructor or a friend to help you up into this pose. Place a folded blanket against the wall. Kneel in front of the blanket with your feet and knees together, and a block between the tops of your thighs. Interlace your fingers firmly, thumbs touching and hands cupped. Position your hands no more than 3 inches from the wall, with your elbows no wider than shoulder-width apart and your wrists perpendicular to the floor (A). Your wrists, forearms, and elbows form the foundation for this pose.

†CAUTION Do this headstand sequence only if it is already part of your yoga practice. Do not do it if you have high blood pressure, are menstruating, or suffer from neck or back problems or migraines.

A

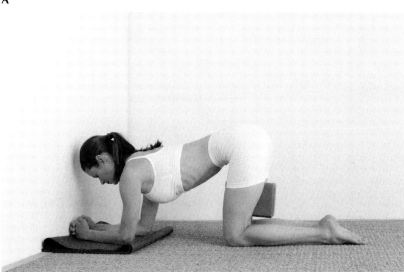

Lengthen your neck and place the crown of your head on the blanket. The back of your head should be in contact with your hands. Press your forearms into the floor and lift your shoulders away from the floor. Maintain this action throughout the pose. As you exhale, bend both legs at once and bring your knees to your chest. Lift your toes off the floor, and slowly move your knees up toward the ceiling (B).

B

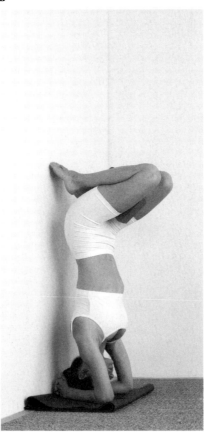

Now stretch your legs straight up. Keep your heels and buttocks against the wall. Roll your thighs in, lift your tailbone, lengthen your legs upward, and keep your feet together. Remember to balance on the crown of your head, support yourself by pressing your forearms into the floor, and continue to lift your shoulders away from your ears. Make sure your anus is slightly higher than your vagina. Keep your breathing even, your eyes and throat soft, and your abdomen relaxed. With practice, you can slowly learn to bring your buttocks and heels away from the wall (C). Remain in this pose for at least a minute but no more than 5 minutes.

C

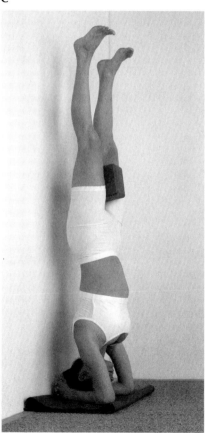

HEADSTAND WITH WIDE-ANGLE LEGS† **(Upavistha Konasana in Sirsasana)**
While in Headstand, have your partner remove the block from between your
legs or slowly come down, remove the block yourself, and return to Headstand
position (see page 89). From Headstand, spread your legs wide, stretching from
your groin through your heels. Keeping your legs straight, stretch up through
your spine and broaden your chest. Remain this way for 10 to 15 seconds.

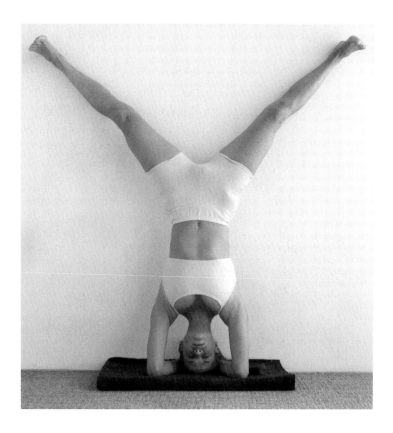

HEADSTAND WITH BOUND ANGLE LEGS† (**Baddha Konasana in Sirsasana**)
From the previous pose, bend your legs, spread your knees outward, and press the soles of your feet together firmly. Remain in this position for another 15 to 20 seconds, keeping your knees wide apart, and breathe normally. Straighten your legs and return to the wide-angle position, then to your original Headstand position.

To come out, exhale and bring your legs down to the floor one at a time. Bend your knees, sit back on your heels, and rest for a few breaths before raising your head.

EFFECTS Using the block "closes" your pelvic region and helps heal any scar tissue. The variations with your legs spread open your pelvis, promote increased circulation to the area, and help ease pain.

†CAUTION Do this headstand sequence only if it is already part of your yoga practice. Do not do it if you have high blood pressure, are menstruating, or suffer from neck or back problems or migraines.

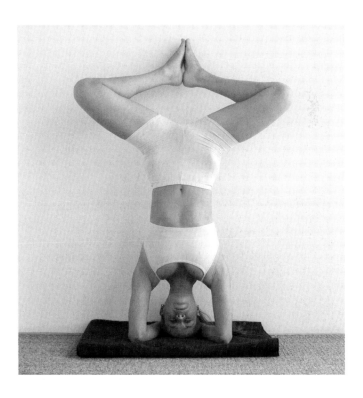

4. LEGS-UP-THE-WALL POSE (Viparita Karani) AND CYCLE† Place a bolster about 3 inches from the wall. (If you are tall, you may need a higher support, such as a folded blanket on top of the bolster.) Sit on the bolster so your right hip and side are touching the wall. Using your hands to support you, lean back and swivel your body around, taking your right leg and then your left leg up the wall. Keep your buttocks close to or against the wall. (If you feel stiffness or discomfort in your legs, push your buttocks slightly away from the wall.) Lie down so your lower back and ribs are supported by the bolster and your shoulders and head are on the floor (A). (If your neck is uncomfortable, put a rolled towel or blanket under it.) Extend through your legs and place your arms out at your sides, elbows bent and palms up. Rest in this position, eyes closed, for 5 minutes.

CYCLE Without moving your torso, allow your legs to open out to the sides (B). Remain in this position, breathing normally, for 3 to 5 minutes.

†CAUTION If menstruating you should not use the bolster with this pose.

A

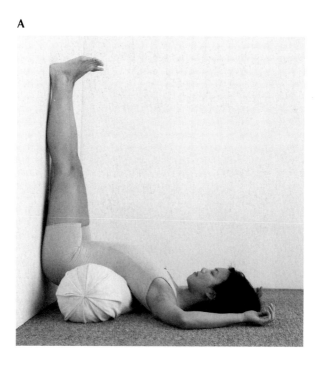

Again keeping your torso in the same position, bend your knees, cross your legs at the ankles, and continue in the pose for another 3 to 5 minutes (C).

B

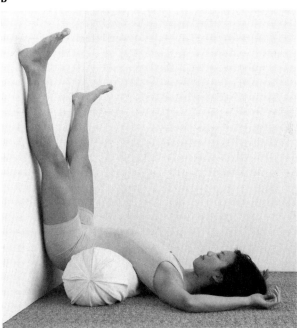

C

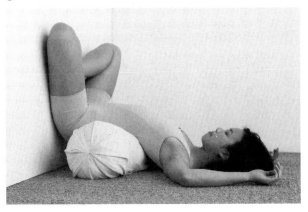

Gently push away from the wall until your buttocks are just off the bolster and resting on the floor; the backs of your thighs and legs remain on the bolster (D). Rest in this position for 5 minutes, or as long as you like.

To come out of the pose, uncross your legs, rest the soles of your feet against the wall, push gently away from the bolster, and roll to one side. Breathe quietly for a few breaths, then use your arms to help you to a seated position.

EFFECTS This deeply restorative pose helps calm the nervous system. It brings breath to the abdomen and "massages" the reproductive organs.

†CAUTION Do not use the bolster with this pose if you are menstruating.

D

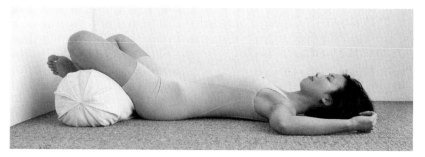

Chapter 7
Uterine Fibroids: Lifestyle Changes Make a Difference

FIBROIDS, OR LEIOMYOMAS AS THEY ARE TECHNICALLY CALLED, affect most women sometime during their reproductive life. In fact, according to the Center for Uterine Fibroids (a division of Brigham and Women's Hospital in Boston), at least 80 percent of all women have these solid masses of muscle and connective tissue lodged in the smooth muscle layer of their uterus (the myometrium). The center also says that the average fibroidal uterus contains six to seven of these benign tumors. Ninety-five percent of all fibroids occur in the uterus. The remaining 5 percent are typically found on the cervix.

Researchers have identified four distinct types of fibroid tumors:

- Subserosal fibroids grow on the outer wall of the uterus. These do not affect menstrual flow; they do, however, cause abdominal cramping and bloating, painful intercourse, and undue pressure on the bladder and bowels.
- Submucosal fibroids grow under the lining of the uterine cavity (the endometrium). These tumors cause heavy bleeding during menstruation, occasionally hemorrhaging as the body attempts to "give birth" to them. Submucosal fibroids are the hardest to treat holistically, but fortunately, they are also the least common.

DIFFERENT TYPES OF
UTERINE FIBROIDS

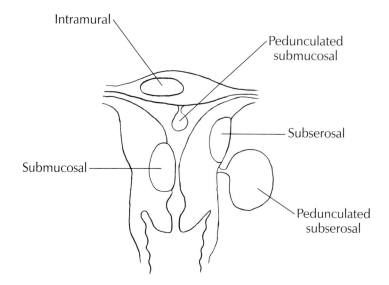

- Intramural fibroids, the most common type, are small growths in the smooth muscle layer of the uterus. Some grow toward the outer wall and develop into subserous growths. Others move toward the endometrium and become submucosal fibroids, which expand and make the uterus feel larger and heavier. Women with intramural fibroids experience heavier than normal menstrual flow, back and pelvic pain, pressure on the bladder, and a frequent need to urinate.

- Pedunculated fibroids grow on a stalk and can live within the uterine walls (submucosal) or attach themselves to the outside of the uterus (subserosal). They often mimic ovarian tumors or cysts, making them difficult to diagnose without exploratory surgery.

WHAT CAUSES UTERINE FIBROIDS?

No one knows exactly what causes fibroids, although theories abound in conventional as well as holistic medicine. Statistics show that African-American women are two to five times more likely than their Caucasian sisters to suffer from fibroids, and women whose mother or sisters have or have had fibroids face a 69 percent likelihood of getting them as well. Overweight women are more susceptible to this type of growth, although plenty of thin women have fibroids too. Oddly enough, smokers are not high-risk candidates. One would think that taking birth control pills would be contraindicated because of their high levels of estrogen (fibroids feed on estrogen), but the Center for Uterine Fibroids contends that oral contraceptives might paradoxically decrease the risk.

So in theory, an overweight, forty-two-year-old, nonsmoking African-American woman who has had several children and whose mother and sisters have the condition is a prime candidate for uterine fibroids. In real life, however, almost all women get fibroids before they reach menopause, but only about 25 to 30 percent experience debilitating symptoms. These include abdominal cramps; pressure on the bladder; heavy bleeding during or between periods; infertility and miscarriages; and frequently, fatigue, indigestion, and constipation. Women whose doctors have identified one fibroid probably have several more that remain undetected.

Fibroids account for more than 250,000 hysterectomies every year—in fact, according to Christiane Northrup, M.D., they are the number-one reason for hysterectomies in this country. They also result in countless prescriptions for pain relievers, which may say more about current medical practice than about the dangers of uterine fibroids. Most fibroids pose little or no problem and shrink considerably once a woman enters menopause. Yet major surgery has been the preferred treatment for many years, particularly for women past their childbearing years.

That said, fibroids can pose potentially serious problems for pregnant women. According to Northrup, that's because hormonal levels soar during pregnancy and fibroids grow rapidly in an estrogen-rich environment.

Risk Factors for Fibroids

- Obesity
- Poor diet (high in fat and low in fiber)
- Too much stress
- Multiple pregnancies
- Family history of fibroids
- Lack of exercise

If the fibroid outgrows its blood supply, it will begin to degenerate or shrink. This degeneration can cause the uterus to contract, which can cause premature delivery. Many women have had successful pregnancies, however, even with moderately large fibroids. Northrup explains that the farther the fibroid is from the uterine cavity, the more likely the woman will have a trouble-free pregnancy.

Most experts agree that estrogen and progesterone have some hand in fibroid growth. Although women with fibroids don't generally have higher levels of estrogen in their bodies, estrogen stimulates fibroid growth. According to the Center for Uterine Fibroids, these tumors may hoard estrogen, have more estrogen receptors, and use it at a faster rate than normal uterine cells. In their book, *Fibroids: The Complete Guide to Taking Charge of Your Physical, Emotional, and Sexual Well-Being*, Johanna Skilling and Eileen Hoffman, M.D., explain that estrogen stimulates a growth hormone called basic fibroblast growth factor. If this hormone gets damaged, it causes muscle cells (of which fibroids are made) to "grow out of control." The fibroids then use the "extra estrogen that they accumulate to make more basic fibroblast growth factor, which in turn helps produce more smooth-muscle cells."

The limited research that exists suggests that progesterone also stimulates fibroid growth. According to observational research done through the Center for Uterine Fibroids, tumors shrink in the presence of RU-386, an antiprogesterone agent. The center also found that fibroids treated with progesterone show "more cellular growth than those from patients without progesterone therapy," and "biochemically, fibroids have higher progesterone receptor concentrations than normal my-ometrium" cells.

Fibroids generally begin to shrink after menopause as the estrogen they depend on decreases. But if you're going through perimenopause with its attendant hormonal fluctuations, your fibroids may grow rapidly. They can also fluctuate in size during your menstrual cycle, growing as you ovulate and then shrinking as you menstruate.

Laura's Story

Laura discovered she had uterine fibroids during a routine exam shortly after her forty-second birthday. Although she had few symptoms (some pressure in her lower abdominals and a heavier-than-normal flow the first two days of her period), her fibroids had grown to the size of golf balls and her uterus had swelled as though she were twenty weeks pregnant. Alarmed at the multiple growths, Laura's gynecologist recommended that she have them removed and possibly undergo a complete hysterectomy. Laura convinced her doctor to give her three to four months to see if lifestyle changes would shrink her fibroids.

With the help of an osteopath specializing in women's health and her yoga teacher, Laura succeeded. She gave up sugar, red meat, and dairy products, and stopped drinking coffee; added essential fatty acids to her diet; and increased her intake of calcium, magnesium, vitamin B complex, and alpha lipoic acid. She got thrice-weekly acupuncture treatments to help her release the feeling of "stuckness" she was experiencing. A daily morning meditation time and afternoon yoga classes relieved her stress levels and gave her an opportunity to breathe life into her reproductive organs. Her osteopath encouraged her to place a hot compress of castor oil on her lower abdomen every other evening before bed as she practiced deep pranayama breathing.

After three months, Laura's doctor declared that the fibroids had shrunk from the size of golf balls to the size of the "bumps on those golf balls."

EMOTIONAL CAUSES OF FIBROIDS

As with most physical conditions, fibroids have an emotional component as well. In many traditions, a woman's uterus is the seat or center of
her creativity, whether that means giving birth to a baby or to ideas, relationships, or herself. In that light, fibroids can often represent those
nonphysical aspects of your being that you can't let go, that you have
trouble releasing into the world. As Laura discovered (see sidebar), her
fibroids disappeared almost completely when yoga afforded her the time
to listen to her body and begin taking care of herself. You may be in a
dead-end job or an unhappy relationship or have trouble communicat-
ing what you really feel. Many women who have been able to let go and
express their true emotions often experience relief.

Ayurvedic physicians believe fibroid tumors stem from chronic imbalances caused by toxins that accumulate in the system and block the
circulation of blood and lymphatic fluids. These blockages prevent nutrients from reaching the tissues and get in the way of the processes that
cleanse the system of impurities. According to the doctors at The Raj, an
ayurvedic treatment center in Fairfield, Iowa, chronic toxin accumulation (ama) in the reproductive tissues "irritate the tissues into responses
that result in the slow accumulation of excess tissue and fibroids." Instead
of surgery, ayurvedic healers use deep tissue massage to open the body's
channels and loosen the impurities so the body can eliminate them.

DIET AND SUPPLEMENTS

What you eat and drink plays an important part in ridding your body of
fibroids, according to both Western and ayurvedic medicine. Western
nutritionists argue for a low-fat (less than 20 grams of fat a day), high-
fiber diet, since high levels of fats and insufficient fiber can lead to increased estrogen levels. They also suggest swearing off alcohol, white
sugar, and all animal products (including dairy, meat, chicken, and fish).
Ayurvedic doctors promote foods that are easy to digest and cleansing
to the system. For the most part, they advise staying away from raw
foods, dairy, meat, and fried foods—anything that's heavy or difficult to

process. They also suggest drinking lots of hot water throughout the day to encourage the downward movement of apana vata (see chapter 3).

Additional B complex vitamins and about 1,000 mg each of methionine, choline, and inositol every day may help break down fibroids. Laura benefited greatly from hot castor oil packs on her abdomen every other night before bed. In addition, therapy or counseling may help uncover any emotional baggage that you need to let go of.

HOW YOGA CAN HELP

Although no studies prove that yoga alone cures or eliminates uterine fibroids, a daily practice coupled with dietary and lifestyle changes can help. Naturally, the earlier you begin yoga, the quicker you'll achieve results. According to Indian author Krishna Raman's book, *A Matter of Health*, the asanas recommended for treatment of fibroids act as an irritant to the reproductive system. That is, these asanas effectively "shut off the blood supply to the fibroid for a short period of time while allowing the blood to flow to other areas."

Inversions do that best. Going upside down virtually "dries out" the uterus and any fibroids growing there, which normally have an ample supply of blood. Twists produce a squeezing and soaking action designed to alternately starve the fibroid and increase blood circulation to the pelvic organs. Patricia says backbends and some standing poses—such as Extended Triangle Pose (Utthita Trikonasana) and Half-Moon Pose (Ardha Chandrasana)—stretch the uterus and relieve congestion in the pelvis. Seated poses such as Bound Angle Pose (Baddha Konasana) and Wide-Angle Seated Pose (Upavistha Konasana) are also beneficial, especially when bleeding is associated with fibroids.

Yogic breathing (pranayama) and the deep relaxation of supported poses such as Reclining Bound Angle Pose (Supta Baddha Konasana) and Corpse Pose (Savasana) move the healing beyond the physical and allow you to spend pressure-free time with your body and mind. Look on it as a chance to discover what feels congested or stuck inside you. This is not the time to judge those feelings; yoga practice simply provides the opportunity to notice them and then let them go.

The sequence Patricia provides here stretches and tones your uterus and reproductive organs, creates space in the pelvis, and in the end provides ample opportunity to completely relax and rejuvenate your body and mind.

A SEQUENCE FOR UTERINE FIBROIDS

1. Reclining Bound Angle Pose (Supta Baddha Konasana)
2. Bound Angle Pose (Baddha Konasana)
3. Wide-Angle Seated Pose I (Upavistha Konasana I)
4. Standing Forward Bend (Uttanasana)
5. Extended Triangle Pose (Utthita Trikonasana)†
6. Half-Moon Pose (Ardha Chandrasana)
7. Headstand (Sirsasana)† or Wide-Angle Standing Forward Bend (Prasarita Padottanasana)†
8. Inverted Staff Pose (Viparita Dandasana)† or Cross Bolsters Pose
9. Child's Pose (Adho Mukha Virasana)
10. Head-on-Knee Pose (Janu Sirsasana)†
11. Simple Seated Twist Pose (Bharadvajasana)†
12. Shoulderstand (Sarvangasana)†
13. Bridge Pose (Setu Bandha Sarvangasana)
14. Legs-Up-the-Wall Pose and Cycle (Viparita Karani)†
15. Corpse Pose (Savasana)

†CAUTION You may want to skip or modify these poses due to health limitations or ability. Please read the explanatory footnote beneath the descriptions before giving them a try.

1. RECLINING BOUND ANGLE POSE (Supta Baddha Konasana) Place a bolster vertically behind you and sit just in front of it with your knees bent and your sacrum touching the bolster's edge. Put a folded blanket on the other end of the bolster to prevent any strain on your neck. Place a strap behind your back, at your sacrum; draw it forward over your hips, across your shins, and under your feet. Put the soles of your feet together and let your knees and thighs release to the sides. Cinch the strap securely under your feet. Lie back so your head is on the folded blanket and your torso rests comfortably on the bolster; your buttocks and legs are on the floor. (If you feel any discomfort in your lower back, add some height to your support with a folded blanket or two. If you feel any muscle tension in your legs, roll two blankets vertically and place one under the top of each thigh.) Take care to relax your abdomen and release your vaginal muscles completely. Breathe evenly and deeply, resting in the pose for at least 5 minutes.

To come out, draw your knees together, slip the strap off, and slowly roll to one side. Use your hands to push yourself up to a seated position.

EFFECTS This deeply relaxing pose helps focus the breath on the abdominal and pelvic organs, which helps massage and tone them.

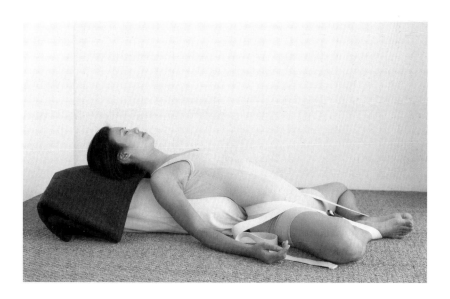

2. BOUND ANGLE POSE (Baddha Konasana) Sit against the wall with your back straight and your abdomen lifted. (If you are menstruating or your hips are tight and you can't lengthen your spine, sit against the wall on a block or blanket about 4 inches thick.) Bending your legs, open your knees out to the sides and bring the soles of your feet together. Hold the tops of your feet and draw your heels in toward your perineum (the pubic bone). The outer edges of your feet should remain on the floor. Lengthen your spine upward, leading with the crown of your head, and release your inner thighs from groin to knee. Place your hands on the floor behind you to sit up straighter, and lift your abdomen. Stay in this position for 30 seconds or more, breathing normally.

To come out, relax your arms and bring your knees up one at a time. Stretch your legs out in front of you.

EFFECTS This is a terrific pose to help alleviate cramps, heavy bleeding, and a feeling of heaviness in your abdomen.

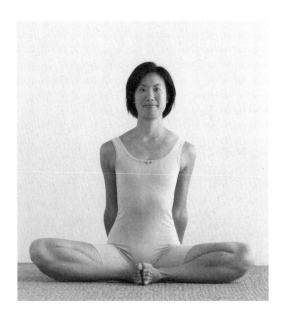

3. WIDE-ANGLE SEATED POSE I (Upavistha Konasana I) Remain against the wall and spread your legs wide apart; extend your ankles and spread and extend your toes. Adjust the flesh of your buttocks by drawing it behind you and out to the sides. If you find it hard to sit up straight in this position, sit on a bolster or the edge of two or more folded blankets positioned against the wall. This helps you sit up on your sitting bones. Place your hands on the floor behind you and moving from the base of your spine, lift and expand your chest. Placing your hands on the floor behind you helps you lengthen up through your lower spine. Sit up tall and press down through your legs. Stay in the pose for 30 seconds to 1 minute. To come out, bend your knees and draw your legs together.

EFFECTS This pose can help the circulation in your pelvic area, regulate your menstrual flow, and stimulate your ovaries.

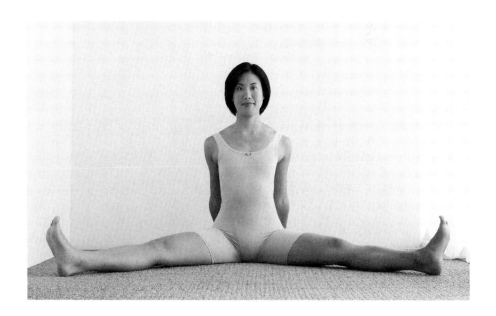

4. STANDING FORWARD BEND (Uttanasana) Place two blocks about shoulder-width apart on the floor in front of you. Stand with your feet together. Stretch your arms over your head. As you exhale, stretch your spine and extend your spine and bend forward from your hips. Place your hands on your blocks and straighten both arms. Lengthen your spine toward your head, lift your head up, and keep your spine concave. Breathe normally for at least 30 to 60 seconds. To come out, place your hands on your hips and lift your torso back to standing position.

EFFECTS This posture will help tone your pelvic floor, improve circulation to your pelvis, and lift and strengthen your uterus.

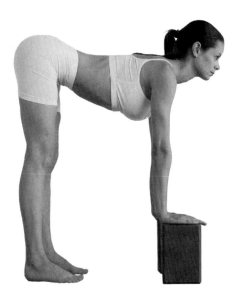

5. EXTENDED TRIANGLE POSE† **(Utthita Trikonasana)** Stand tall with your legs together or slightly apart. Step your feet about 3½ feet apart; turn your left foot out 90 degrees and your right foot slightly inward. The heel of your left foot should line up with the arch of your right. (Place a block beside the outside edge of your left foot if you need to.) Stretch your arms out to the sides, draw up through your quadriceps, and lift your abdomen and chest. On an exhalation, keeping your back straight, extend your trunk to the left and bring your left hand down to the floor or the block. Press your hand into the floor or block, lengthen your spine and expand your chest, and stretch your right arm

†CAUTION If you feel fatigued or experience bleeding with your fibroids, either skip this pose or use the wall to support your head and back.

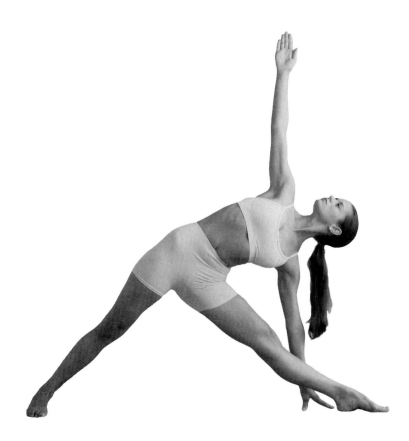

toward the ceiling. Draw your shoulder blades in, turn your chest and abdomen toward the ceiling, and look straight ahead or up at your right hand. Breathe normally for 20 to 30 seconds. To come out, press down through your right heel and inhale as you stretch up through your left arm. Repeat the pose on your right side before returning to a standing position.

EFFECTS Because of the deep twisting action of this pose, it helps balance your liver, kidney, and spleen function; increases blood flow to your pelvic region; and tones and improves the function of your reproductive and digestive organs. It can also help relieve anxiety and nervous tension.

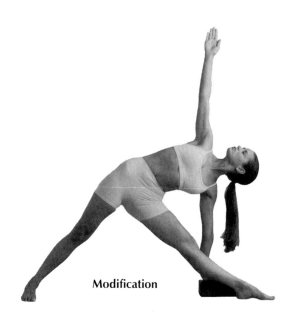

Modification

6. HALF-MOON POSE (Ardha Chandrasana) Begin in Triangle Pose (Utthita Trikonasana) (A): Stand up tall with your back close to the wall. Step your feet as wide as possible, at least 3 to 4 feet apart, and place a block near your left foot. Turn your left foot out 90 degrees and your right foot slightly inward. The heel of your left foot should line up with the arch of your right. Stretch your arms out to the sides, draw up through your quadriceps, and lift your abdomen and chest. On an exhalation, keeping your back straight, extend your trunk to the left and bring your left hand down to the block (A). Bend your left knee, pick up the block with the fingertips of your left hand and move it about a foot in front of your left leg against the wall. Come up onto the toes of your left foot. Exhale, simultaneously straightening your left leg and raising your right until it is parallel to the floor. Your right leg, hips, shoulders, and head should rest against the wall. Turn your pelvis and chest toward the ceiling. Stretch your right arm up in

A

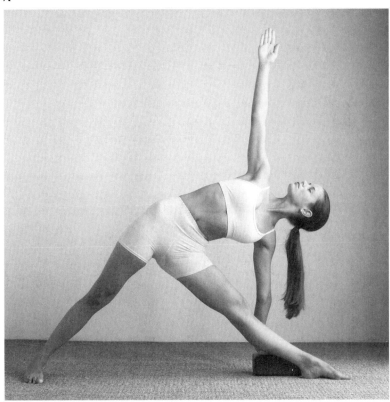

line with your shoulders and open your chest and pelvis farther. Draw your shoulder blades into your back and look up at your right hand or straight ahead (B). Hold for 15 seconds, breathing normally.

To come out, bend your left leg, reach back through your right leg, and place your right foot on the floor, returning to Extended Triangle Pose. Inhale, come to standing, and repeat on the other side. End in a standing position with your feet together.

EFFECTS This pose is particularly advantageous if you have backaches as well as abdominal cramps. The wall allows you to rest completely and not worry about holding yourself up. This pose also helps you relax your abdomen and vaginal muscles fully so you can breathe deeply into that part of your body. Gripping these muscles can create stagnation in your reproductive organs.

B

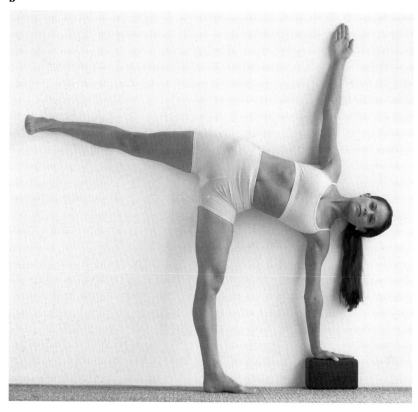

7. HEADSTAND† **(Sirsasana)** Place a folded blanket against the wall. Kneel in front of it with your feet and knees together. Interlace your fingers firmly, thumbs touching and hands cupped. Position your hands no more than 3 inches from the wall, your elbows shoulder-width apart. Your wrists, forearms, and elbows form the foundation for this pose.

Lengthen your neck and place the crown of your head on the blanket. The back of your head should be in contact with your hands. Press your forearms into the floor and lift your shoulders away from the floor. Maintain this action throughout the pose. Straighten your legs, raise your hips toward the ceiling, and walk your feet in until your spine is almost per-pendicular to the floor. As you exhale, lift one leg at a time, and bring your feet to the wall.

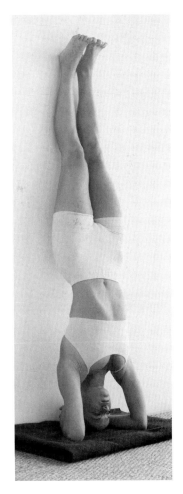

Keep your heels and buttocks against the wall. Lengthen up through your inner legs and inner heels, and keep your feet together. Remember to balance on the crown of your head, support your-self by pressing your forearms into the floor, and continue to lift your shoulders away from your ears. Keep your breathing even, your eyes and throat soft, and your abdomen relaxed. With regular prac-tice, you can slowly learn to bring your buttocks and heels away from the wall. Hold the pose as long as you can, up to 5 minutes.

EFFECTS This rejuvenating headstand sequence is excellent for rebalancing your endocrine system to get it ready for your next cycle. It also increases cir-culation in your pelvis and tones your uterus.

†CAUTION Do this sequence only if it is already part of your yoga practice. Seek the advice of an experi-enced teacher if you have neck problems. Do not do this sequence if you are menstruating or suffer from back problems or migraines.

HEADSTAND WITH WIDE-ANGLE LEGS (Upavistha Konasana in Sirsasana)
Before trying these next two poses, you need to be comfortable remaining in
Headstand for 3 to 5 minutes. From Headstand, spread your legs wide, stretching from your groin through your heels. Keeping your legs straight, stretch
up through your spine and broaden your chest. Remain this way for 10 to 15
seconds.

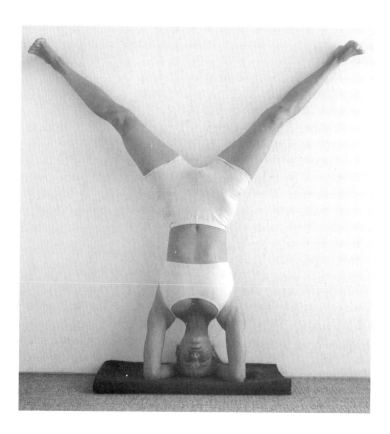

HEADSTAND WITH BOUND ANGLE LEGS (Baddha Konasana in Sirsasana)
From the previous pose, bend your legs, spread your knees outward, and press the soles of your feet together firmly. Remain in this position for another 15 to 20 seconds, keeping your knees wide apart, and breathe normally. Straighten your legs and return to the wide-angle position, then to your original Headstand position.

To come out, exhale and bring your legs down to the floor one at a time. Bend your knees, sit back on your heels, and rest for a few breaths before raising your head.

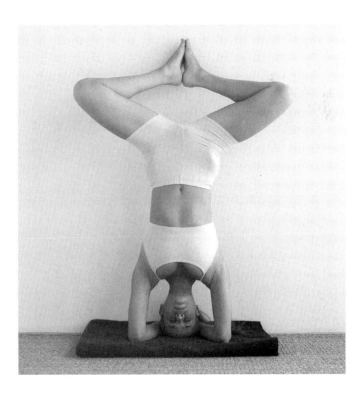

ALTERNATIVE: WIDE-ANGLE STANDING FORWARD BEND† (Prasarita Padot-tanasana) If Headstand is not part of your normal practice, this pose offers many of the same benefits. Step your feet apart about 4 feet (or as wide as possible), keeping the outer edges of your feet parallel. Tighten your quadriceps to draw your kneecaps up and keep your thighs well lifted. On an exhalation, bend forward from your hips and place your hands on the floor, underneath your shoulders and straighten your arms (A). (If you feel strain in your lower back, place your hands on blocks.) Lift your hips toward the ceiling, draw your inner back thighs away from each other as you lengthen your spine forward (toward your head). Move your shoulder blades into your back and look up. Your mid- to upper-thoracic spine will be slightly concave. Remain this way for 10 to 25 seconds.

A

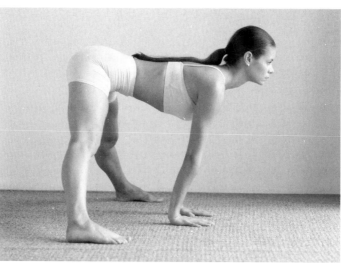

Keeping your trunk extended, exhale, bend your elbows, and release the crown of your head down and place your hands on the floor, if possible (B). Keep your legs firm, but relax your shoulders and neck. Breathe deeply and let your trunk release downward. Stay in this pose for 30 to 60 seconds.

To come out, bring your hands to your hips, return to the concave back position, and raise your trunk. Step your feet together.

EFFECTS Overall, both variations will increase circulation in the pelvic region and help restore equilibrium to your endocrine system, so necessary for a healthy cycle.

†CAUTION Do not do the second part of this pose (B) if you suffer from low blood pressure or have low energy associated with a drop in blood sugar.

B

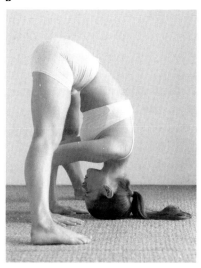

8. INVERTED STAFF POSE† **(Viparita Dandasana)** Place a folded blanket on a chair about 2 feet from the wall—far enough away so your feet can press into the wall when your legs are outstretched. Pile two bolsters against the wall for your feet, and put a bolster (and a folded blanket, if necessary) in front of the chair for your head. Sit facing the wall, with your feet through the chair back. Hold on to the sides of the chair and support yourself on your elbows, as you arch back slowly. Your head, neck, and shoulders should extend past the chair seat and your shoulder blades should touch the front edge of the seat.

Still holding the sides of the chair, arch back so your shoulder blades are at the front edge of the seat and your head can rest on its support. (You may need to scoot your buttocks farther toward the back of the seat.) Put your feet on top of the bolsters and against the wall, legs slightly bent, and hold the back legs or sides of the chair. Straighten your legs, pressing your feet into the wall, and roll your thighs in toward each other. Rest your head on the bolster. Keep your hands on the chair sides or legs. Breathe quietly for 30 to 60 seconds.

To come out, bend your knees and place your feet flat on the floor. Grasp the sides of the chair back and lift up from your sternum. Lean over the chair back for a few breaths to release your back.

EFFECTS This pose stretches your uterus, acting as an irritant to fibroids and working to starve them of blood.

†CAUTION Do not do this pose if you have neck problems or headaches.

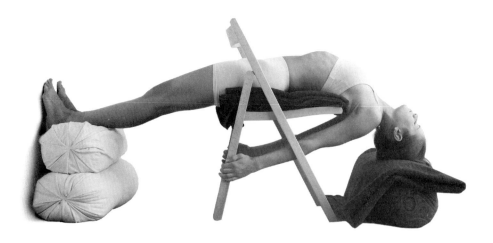

ALTERNATIVE: CROSS BOLSTERS POSE Place a bolster on your mat and lay another one across the center of the first to form a cross. Sit on the middle of the top bolster and carefully lie back so your spine is supported on the bolster and the back of your head touches the floor. (If that is too much of a stretch or puts strain on your neck, place a folded blanket underneath your head.) Place your arms on either side of your head, palms up, elbows bent, and relax completely. (If you feel any strain in your lower back, raise your feet on a block.) Relax in this pose for several minutes, softening your abdominal muscles and breathing deeply.

To come out of the pose, bend your knees and roll to one side. Help yourself up using your hands.

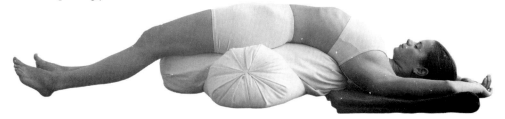

9. CHILD'S POSE (Adho Mukha Virasana) Kneel on the floor with your knees slightly wider than your hips and bring your big toes together. Bend forward and stretch your arms and trunk forward. Rest your head on the floor or a blanket.

EFFECTS This pose calms your nervous system and is a nice counterpose to any backbends.

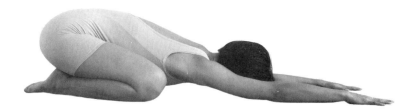

10. HEAD-ON-KNEE POSE† **(Janu Sirsasana)** Sit on the floor with your legs stretched out in front of you. (If you can't sit up tall without rounding your back, sit on a bolster or two folded blankets.) Bend your right knee to the side and place your right foot against the inside of your left thigh. Keep your left leg straight.

Turn your abdomen and chest so your sternum is in line with the center of your left leg. With an exhalation, bend forward from your hips and catch the sides of your left foot with your hands; straighten your arms. Inhale as you lift from the base of your spine and move it up and in (spine should be concave). Keep your head and back lifted (A). (If this is difficult to do without bending your left knee, use a strap looped around the ball of your foot.) Remain in this pose for 15 to 20 seconds, if possible.

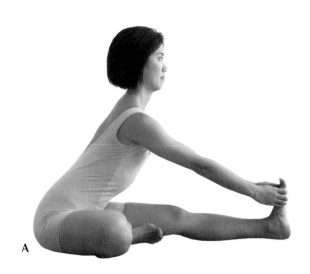

A

Exhale and bend your arms to come forward as you length your spine toward your foot. Rest your head on your left shin without straining (B). If you can't reach your head to your shin, lengthen your spine toward your foot and bring your head down onto a bolster placed aross your shin (see page 14). Stay in this pose for 30 seconds, resting your head, the base of your skull, your eyes, and your mind.

To come out, lift your head and torso slightly, release your hands, and sit up. Straighten your right leg, and repeat the pose on the other side.

EFFECTS This pose counteracts the effects of stress on your body and mind and relieves stiffness in your hips and sacrum area. In addition, because of its twisting action, it has a toning and activating effect on your liver, spleen, kidneys, and reproductive organs.

†CAUTION Do not do this pose if you have diarrhea or sciatica.

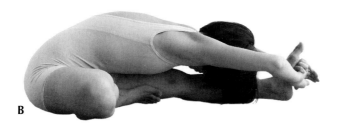

B

11. SIMPLE SEATED TWIST POSE† **(Bharadvajasana)** Sit up straight with your legs stretched out in front of you and your left hip elevated on a folded blanket or two. Bend both legs to the right so your feet are next to your right hip. Keeping your thighs and knees facing forward, make sure your right ankle rests on the arch of your left foot and that your buttocks are not on top of your foot. Draw your shoulder blades into your back, broaden your chest, and extend your spine upward. On an exhalation, turn your abdomen, ribs, chest, and shoulders (in that order) to the left; place your right hand on the outside of your left thigh and your left hand on the floor behind you (or on a block). Take several breaths, holding the posture for 20 to 30 seconds. Relax your face, neck, and throat. Come back to the center position, straighten your legs, and change sides.

EFFECTS The gentle twist in this pose massages your reproductive organs, energizes your adrenal glands, and tones your kidneys.

†CAUTION Do not practice twists if you have diarrhea or feel nausea. Do not do this pose if you have arthritis in your knees. If you suffer from sacroiliac pain, release your pelvis whenever you twist.

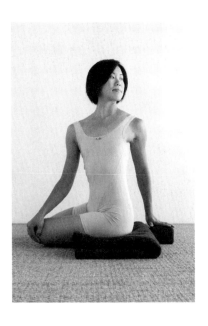

12. SHOULDERSTAND† **(Sarvangasana)** Place a chair about 8 to 10 inches away from the wall. Put a folded blanket on the chair seat, and two or three folded blankets in front of the chair. Sit backward on the chair with your legs bent over the top of the back; move your buttocks into the center of the chair seat (A).

†CAUTION Do not do this pose if you suffer from neck or shoulder problems, if you are menstruating, or if you have a migraine or tension headache.

A

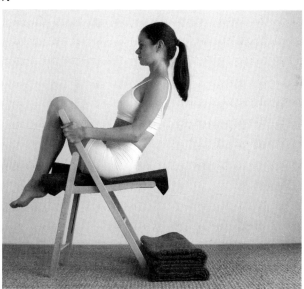

B

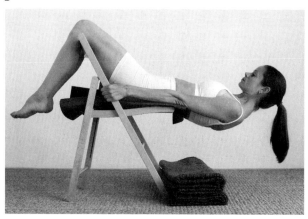

Holding the sides and then the front legs of the chair, slowly lower your torso so your shoulders are on the blankets and your head is on the floor (B). You must extend your spine and open your chest while doing this to get the proper position. Move your hands, one at a time, to hold the back legs of the chair; your arms should be between the front legs (C). Stretch your legs straight up, keeping your sacrum on the chair seat. Rotate your thighs in and extend from your groin to your heels. Close your eyes, bring your chest to your chin (D), and breathe normally for 3 to 5 minutes, or as long as you're comfortable.

To release from the pose, bend your knees and place your feet on the chair back (E). Release your hands, and slide down until your sacrum rests on the blankets and your calves are on the chair seat. Rest here a moment, then roll to your side and sit up slowly.

EFFECTS This pose has been known to balance the thyroid and parathyroid glands and help ease uterine dysplasia associated with fibroids.

C

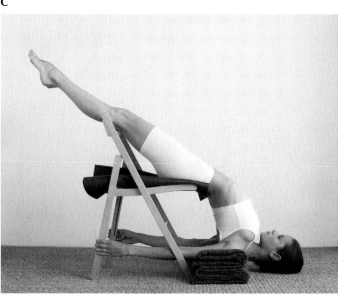

D

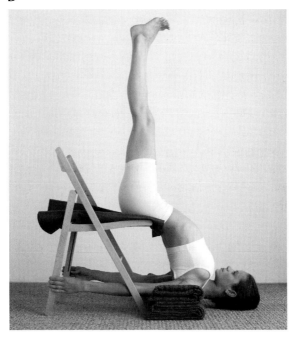

E

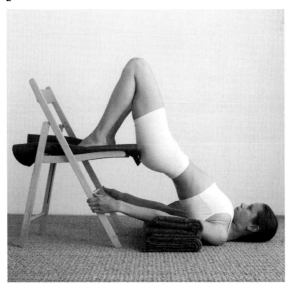

13. BRIDGE POSE (Setu Bandha Sarvangasana) Place a block vertically against the wall and have another at your side. Lie on your back with your arms at your sides and your knees bent. Raise your hips and chest as high as possible and support your back with your hands. Keeping your head and shoulders flat on the floor, lift your spine even farther, increasing the arch, and place the other vertical block under the fleshy part of your buttocks. Stretch out one leg at a time, resting each heel on the vertical block against the wall. Release your arms so that your hands reach just beyond the block under your sacrum. Hold the pose for at least 30 seconds, breathing normally.

To come out, bend your knees and place your feet on the floor. Then release the block under your sacrum and slowly roll down one vertebra at a time. Hug both knees to your chest and rest for several breaths.

EFFECTS This slightly more active pose tones and improves circulation to your kidneys and adrenal glands, which is very important to good reproductive health. If you feel irritable or fatigued, try the modification shown below.

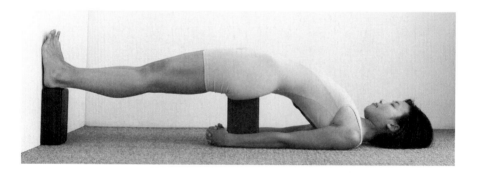

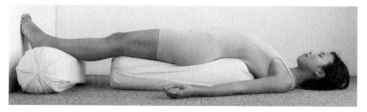

Modification

14. LEGS-UP-THE-WALL CYCLE (Viparita Karani) AND CYCLE† Place a bolster about 3 inches from the wall. (If you are tall, you may need a higher support, such as a folded blanket on top of the bolster.) Sit on the bolster so your right hip and side are touching the wall. Using your hands to support you, lean back and swivel your body around, taking your right leg and then your left leg up the wall. Keep your buttocks close to or against the wall. (If you feel stiffness or discomfort in your legs, push your buttocks slightly away from the wall.) Lie down so your lower back and ribs are supported by the bolster and your shoulders and head are on the floor (A). (If your neck is uncomfortable, put a rolled towel or blanket under it.) Extend through your legs and place your arms out at your sides, elbows bent and palms up. Rest in this position, eyes closed, for 5 minutes.

†CAUTION Do not use the bolster with this pose if you are menstruating.

A

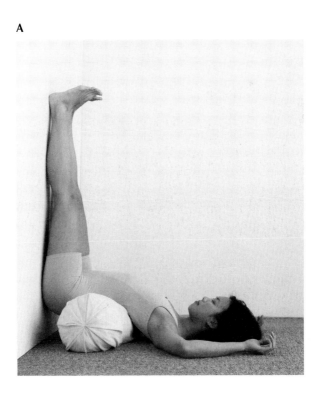

CYCLE Without moving your torso, allow your legs to open out to the sides (B). Remain in this position, breathing normally, for 3 to 5 minutes.

Again keeping your torso in the same position, bend your knees, cross your legs at the ankles, and continue in the pose for another 3 to 5 minutes (C).

Gently push away from the wall until your buttocks are just off the bolster and resting on the floor; the backs of your thighs and legs remain on the bolster (D). Rest in this position for 5 minutes, or as long as you like.

To come out of the pose, uncross your legs, rest the soles of your feet against the wall, and gently push away from the bolster, and roll to one side. Breathe quietly for a few breaths, then use your arms to help you to a seated position.

B

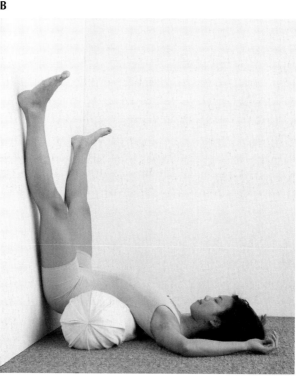

EFFECTS This deeply restorative pose calms your sympathetic nervous system and helps relax your abdomen and pelvic floor muscles so healing of fibroids can begin.

C

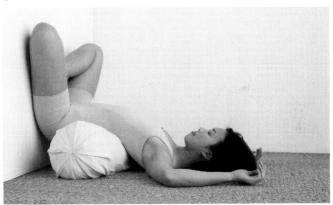

D

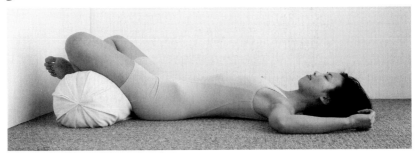

15. CORPSE POSE (Savasana) Lie on your back with your legs stretched out in front of you and your eyes closed completely. (Use a folded blanket to support your head, if necessary.) Place your arms comfortably at your sides, slightly away from your torso, with your palms facing upward. Actively stretch your arms and legs away from you and then allow them to release completely. With soft inhalations and quiet exhalations, surrender your body to the floor, without tensing your throat, neck, or diaphragm. Sense that your muscles are releasing from the bones and your skin is releasing from the muscles. Relax your eyes, ears, facial skin, and tongue and, as you exhale, feel your external organs resting against your back body. Keep your abdomen soft and relaxed, and release your lower back. Spread your awareness—your mind—through your body and let it come to rest in the heart. Remain in the pose, breathing normally, for 5 to 10 minutes. To come out, bend your knees, roll to one side, remain there for a few breaths, and then open your eyes and push yourself up with your hands.

EFFECTS This pose will further soothe your sympathetic nervous system, rejuvenate your whole body, and help your body integrate the benefits of the other poses.

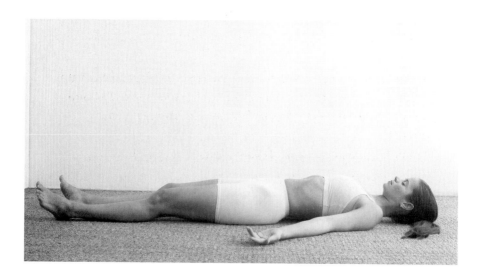

Chapter 8
Back to Normal: Postmenstruation

ONCE YOUR PERIOD IS OVER, YOU'RE PROBABLY EAGER TO RETURN to your normal routine, including your daily yoga practice. Patricia believes you shouldn't rush things. Your body needs to regain strength and stamina. We've provided several poses at the end of the chapter that you'll find beneficial for the first three to five days after you stop bleeding. In the meantime, keep the following dos and don'ts in mind:

- Don't do backbends right away—they're too aggressive. Allow your body to recover from the fatigue of your monthly cycle first.

- Do incorporate inversions immediately because they help dry up your uterus, restore your endocrine system, increase circulation to your abdominal region, and help your body regain its strength.

- Don't do a lot of standing poses the first couple of days if you still feel fatigue. Ease into them.

STAYING HEALTHY ALL MONTH LONG

The most important thing you can do to minimize menstrual problems is to take care of your body and honor yourself every day. If you know, for example, that drinking coffee or soda brings on premenstrual headaches, find a decaffeinated substitute. By avoiding greasy foods and sugary desserts, cutting down on alcohol and caffeinated beverages, and substituting home-cooked meals for processed foods, you may find much of your physical and emotional discomfort goes away. Here are some other suggestions many women have found helpful.

- *Get sufficient rest.* If you do nothing else for yourself, rest during the first day or two of your period. You'll be amazed at how much better you feel the rest of the month. This doesn't mean you should sleep during the day—that can make you feel sluggish and depressed. It does mean you should relax, read that book you've been meaning to get to, take walks with no particular place to go. If you have children, find quiet activities you can do together. If you have to go to school or work, be easy on yourself, schedule a lighter-than-usual load, and take the evening off.

- *Be selfish.* The first day or two of your period is a time for reflection. If you meditate, now is a good time to practice loving kindness toward yourself, your family, and your friends. Do things that make you feel good about being you.

- *Exercise in moderation.* Unless you are plagued with debilitating cramps the first day of your period, exercise is fine; just don't overdo it. Walking or gentle yoga stretches (see the healthy menstruation sequence in chapter 2) work best. During the rest of the month, a consistent yoga practice and moderate aerobic exercise should help prevent premenstrual syndrome (PMS) and menstrual problems from occurring in the first place.

- *Eat pacifying foods.* During the first day or two of your cycle, eat warm foods that are easy to digest, such as rice, cooked green vegetables, and soups. Avoid cold, raw foods, as well as anything else that's hard to digest, such as red meat, cheese, and chocolate. Sip warm water throughout the day to aid digestion.

- *Take your vitamins.* Calcium, magnesium, and vitamin D are all useful for women at any time during their cycle. Some studies suggest that PMS may actually be synonymous with hypocalcemia (calcium deficiency). Researchers have found that calcium levels drop just before your period as estrogen levels increase. If you are low in calcium to begin with, you may experience fatigue, depression, anxiety, fuzzy thinking, irritability, or cramping before your period starts. Be sure you get at least 1,500 mg of calcium daily, through a variety of sources—green vegetables, fruits, soy, dairy, supplements—and half as much magnesium. Do not, however, take more than 500 mg of a calcium supplement at a time. Your body can't absorb more than that. Instead, take 500 mg in the morning and 500 mg at night.

- *Modify your routine.* Baths disrupt the natural rhythm of your menstrual flow, so shower the first few days of your period. After that, treat yourself to a warm oil massage or a facial to destress your nervous system and soothe your mind. Whenever you can, wear menstrual pads rather than tampons, especially during the first few days of your period, to encourage the downward flow of blood.

A SEQUENCE FOR POSTMENSTRUATION

1. Downward-Facing Dog Pose (Adho Mukha Svanasana)
2. Standing Forward Bend (Uttanasana)
3. Wide-Angle Standing Forward Bend (Prasarita Padottanasana)†
4. Headstand (Sirsasana)†
5. Shoulderstand (Sarvangasana)†
6. Plough Pose (Halasana)†
7. Head-on-Knee Pose (Janu Sirsasana)
8. Corpse Pose (Savasana)

†CAUTION You may want to skip or modify these poses due to health limitations or ability. Please read the explanatory footnote beneath the descriptions before giving them a try.

1. DOWNWARD-FACING DOG POSE (Adho Mukha Svanasana) To find the correct distance between your hands and feet for this pose, lie facedown on your sticky mat. Place your palms on the floor by each side of your chest with your fingers well spread and pointing straight ahead. Come up on your hands and knees, and turn your toes under. (If you feel tired or stiff, rest your head on a bolster or folded blanket.)

Exhale, press your hands firmly into the mat, and extend up through your inner arms. Exhale again as you raise your buttocks high in the air and move your thighs up and back. Keep stretching through your legs and bring your heels toward the floor. Keep your legs firm and your elbows straight as you lift your buttocks upward. The action of your arms and legs serves to elongate your spine and release your head. Hold this pose for 30 seconds to 1 minute, breathing deeply. Let your head rest completely and release the base of your neck. To come out, either return to your hands and knees and sit back on your heels.

EFFECTS This pose helps increase the blood supply to your brain and enhance circulation in your chest.

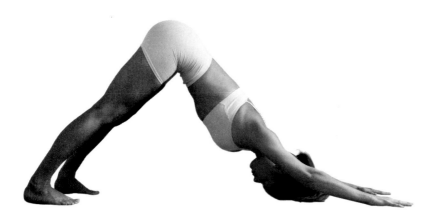

2. STANDING FORWARD BEND (Uttanasana) Stand with your feet together or slightly apart. Distribute your weight evenly between your feet, lengthen up through your inner thighs, and roll your thighs in. Keep your legs and knees firm as you lift your arms overhead, stretching up through your waist and ribs. As you exhale, bend forward from your hips and release your side body and head down toward your knees. Press your hands into the floor next to your feet. (If you can't touch the floor, rest your hands on blocks or on your shins.) Breathe normally for 30 to 60 seconds. To come out, keep your legs active, put your hands on your hips, and slowly lift up to standing.

EFFECTS This pose brings a sense of calm and peace when you feel agitated or anxious. It also tones your liver, spleen, and kidneys and lifts and tones your uterus.

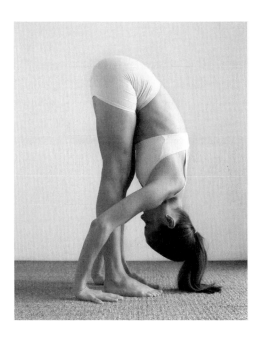

3. WIDE-ANGLE STANDING FORWARD BEND† (Prasarita Padottanasana) Step your feet apart about 4 feet (or as wide as possible), keeping the outer edges of your feet parallel to your mat. Tighten your quadriceps to draw your kneecaps up and keep your thighs well lifted. On an exhalation, bend forward from your hips and place your hands on the floor, in line with your shoulders (A). (If you feel strain in your lower back, place your hands on blocks.) Lift your hips toward the ceiling, draw your shoulder blades into your back, and look up, keeping your entire spine concave. Remain this way for 10 to 15 seconds.

Keeping your trunk extended, exhale, bend your elbows, and release the crown of your head toward the floor—resting it on the floor, if possible (B).

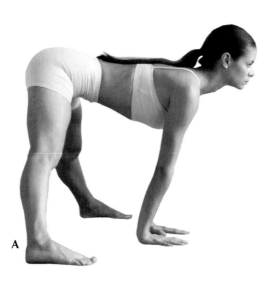

A

Keep your legs firm, but relax your shoulders and neck. Breathe deeply and let your trunk release downward. Stay in this pose for 30 to 60 seconds.

To come out, return to the concave back position, bring your hands to your hips, and raise your trunk. Step your feet together.

EFFECTS This pose can be helpful when you're trying to combat fatigue, calm your mind, tone your abdominal region, and soothe jittery nerves. It also lifts your uterus, improves circulation in your pelvis, and helps restore equilibrium to your central nervous system.

†CAUTION Do not do the B part of the pose if you suffer from low blood pressure or have low energy associated with a drop in blood sugar.

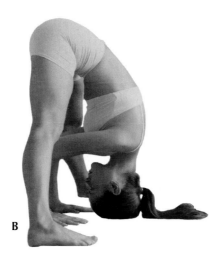

B

4. HEADSTAND† **(Sirsasana)** Place a folded blanket against the wall. Kneel in front of it with your feet and knees together. Interlace your fingers firmly, thumbs touching and hands cupped (A). Position your hands no more than 3 inches from the wall, your elbows shoulder-width apart. Your wrists, forearms, and elbows form the foundation for this pose.

Lengthen your neck and place the crown of your head on the blanket. The back of your head should be in contact with your hands. Press your forearms into the floor and lift your shoulders away from the floor. Maintain this action throughout the pose. Straighten your legs, raise your hips toward the ceiling, and walk your feet in until your spine is almost perpendicular to the floor. As you exhale, lift one leg at a time, and bring your feet to the wall (B).

Keep your heels and buttocks against the wall. Lengthen up through your inner legs and inner heels, and keep your feet together (C). Remember to balance

C

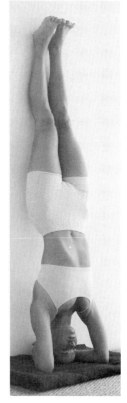

B

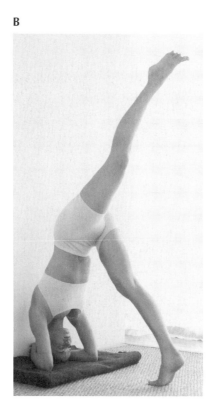

A

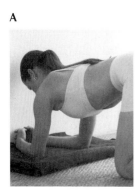

on the crown of your head, support yourself by pressing your forearms into the floor, and continue to lift your shoulders away from your ears. Keep your breathing even, your eyes and throat soft, and your abdomen relaxed. With regular practice, you can slowly learn to bring your buttocks and heels away from the wall. Hold the pose as long as you can, up to 5 minutes. Move on to the following two poses only if you are comfortable in Headstand for 3 to 5 minutes.

HEADSTAND WITH WIDE-ANGLE LEGS (Upavistha Konasana in Sirsasana)
From Headstand, spread your legs wide, stretching from your groin through your heels. Keeping your legs straight, stretch up through your spine and broaden your chest. Remain this way for 10 to 15 seconds.

†CAUTION Do these poses only if they are already part of your yoga practice. Seek the advice of an experienced teacher if you have neck problems. Do not do these poses if you suffer from back problems or migraines.

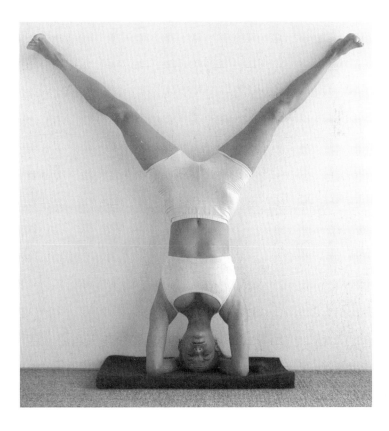

HEADSTAND WITH BOUND ANGLE LEGS† (**Baddha Konasana in Sirsasana**)
From the previous pose, bend your legs, spread your knees outward, and press the soles of your feet together firmly. Remain in this position for another 15 to 20 seconds, keeping your knees wide apart, and breathe normally. Straighten your legs and return to the wide-angle position, then to your original Headstand position.

To come out, exhale and bring your legs down to the floor one at a time. Bend your knees, sit back on your heels, and rest for a few breaths before raising your head.

EFFECTS This rejuvenating pose is excellent for rebalancing your endocrine system to get it ready for your next cycle. This three-part pose also increases circulation in your pelvis and tones your uterus.

†CAUTION Do these poses only if they are already part of your yoga practice. Seek the advice of an experienced teacher if you have neck problems. Do not do these poses if you suffer from back problems or migraines.

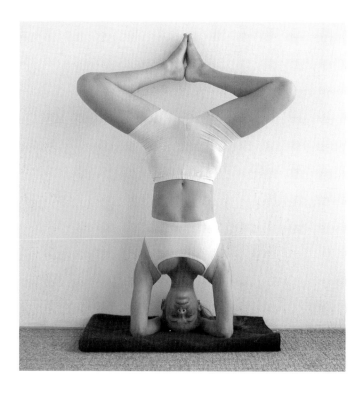

5. SHOULDERSTAND† **(Sarvangasana)** If this unsupported version of Shoulderstand is too difficult, do the modified version using a chair (see chapter 5). Lie on your back with two folded blankets supporting your shoulders with your arms outstretched beside you. On an exhalation, bend your knees and raise your legs toward your chest. Pressing your hands into the floor, swing your bent legs over your head; support your back with your hands and press your elbows firmly into the blankets. Raise your torso up until it is perpendicular to the floor and your knees are close to your chest (A). Supporting your back, raise your legs until your thighs are parallel to the floor (B); raise them some more until your

†CAUTION Do not do this pose if you suffer from neck or shoulder problems, if you have high blood pressure, or if you have a migraine or tension headache.

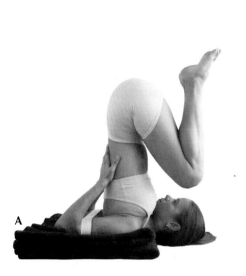

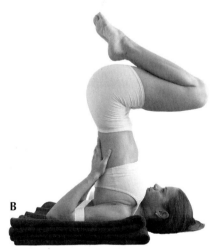

A B

knees point toward the ceiling (C). Now raise your legs completely and extend up through your heels until your whole body is perpendicular to the floor. Move your tailbone up and in and use your hands to lift your back ribs (D). Feel that your whole body is long and straight. Move your shoulders away from your ears. Hold this pose as long as you can, preferably at least 2 minutes.

To come out, exhale as you bend your knees. Slowly roll down. Lie still for several breaths.

EFFECTS This pose may help improve thyroid and parathyroid function, which is vital for good menstrual health. It soothes your nerves, stimulates your kidneys, and calms your mind, bringing a sense of peace, strength, and new resolve if you still feel fatigued after your period is over.

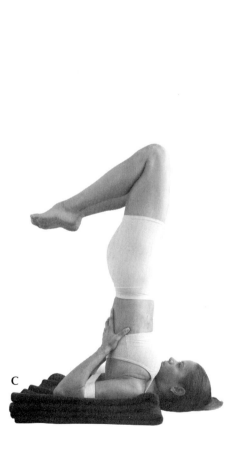

C

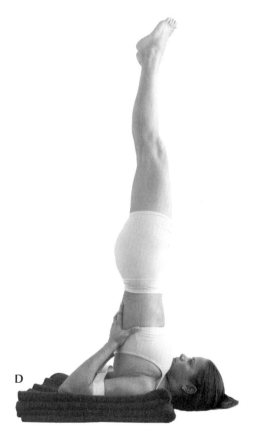

D

6. PLOUGH POSE† (Halasana) Lie on your back with two folded blankets supporting your shoulders; your head is on the sticky mat and your arms are down by your sides, palms pressed into the floor. (If you have trouble keeping your elbows from splaying apart, secure a strap around your arms, just above the elbows.) Bend your knees and bring your thighs in to your chest. On an exhalation, swing or lift your buttocks and legs up, supporting your back with your hands, and extend your legs over your head, placing your toes on the floor behind you. Keep your elbows in toward one another. Move your inner thighs up toward the ceiling and extend your calves to the heels to create space between your face and your legs. Stay in this pose, breathing deeply and slowly, for several minutes.

To come out, slowly roll down one vertebra at a time. Rest with your back flat on the floor, breathing deeply, for several breaths. If this pose is too difficult, try Half-Plough Pose (Ardha Halasana) as described on page 71.

EFFECTS This pose helps balance your endocrine system and quiet your sympathetic nervous system. Resting this way can help tame irritability and anxiety. It also tones your abdominal organs, elongates and strengthens your spine, and relieves fatigue.

†CAUTION Do not do this pose if you have neck problems.

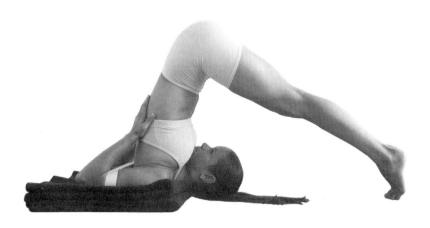

7. HEAD-ON-KNEE POSE (Janu Sirsasana) Sit with your legs stretched out in front of you. (If you can't sit without rounding your back, sit up on a bolster or two folded blankets.) Bend your right knee to the side and place your right foot against the inside of your left thigh. Loop a strap around the ball of your left foot and then straighten your left leg. (If you are flexible enough, you may catch the sides of your left foot with both hands.)

Turn your abdomen and chest to the left so your sternum is in line with the center of your left leg. With an exhalation, bend forward from your hips and

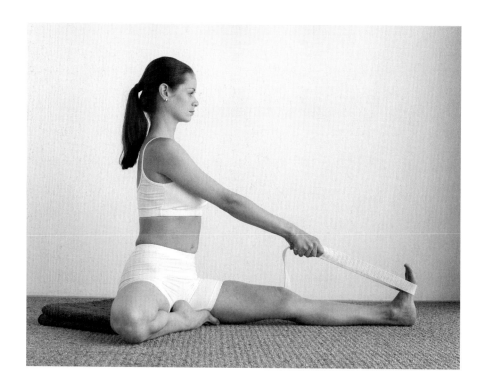

pull back on the strap (or your foot), straightening both arms; keep your head and back lifted. Inhale as you lift from the base of your spine and move it up and in. (Your spine should be concave.) Remain like this for 15 to 20 seconds, if possible. To come out, release your hands on the strap and straighten your right foot. Repeat the pose on the other side.

EFFECTS Because of the gentle twist, this pose has a toning effect on your reproductive organs and the supporting muscles.

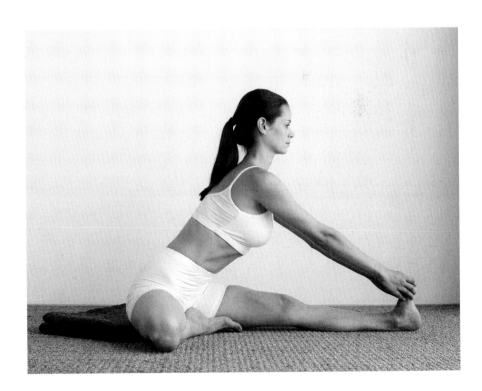

8. CORPSE POSE (Savasana) Lie on your back with your legs stretched out in front of you and your eyes closed completely. (Use a folded blanket to support your head, if necessary.) Place your arms comfortably at your sides, slightly away from your torso, with your palms facing upward. Actively stretch your arms and legs away from you and then allow them to release completely. With soft inhalations and quiet exhalations, surrender your body to the floor, without tensing your throat, neck, or diaphragm. Sense that your muscles are releasing from the bones and your skin is releasing from the muscles. Relax your eyes, ears, facial skin, and tongue and, as you exhale, feel your external organs resting against your back body. Keep your abdomen soft and relaxed, and release your lower back. Spread your awareness—your mind—through your body and let it come to rest in the heart. Remain in the pose, breathing normally, for 5 to 10 minutes. To come out, bend your knees, roll to one side, remain there for a few breaths, and then open your eyes and push yourself up with your hands.

EFFECTS This restorative pose helps relax your mind, quiet your nervous system, and refresh and invigorate your whole body.

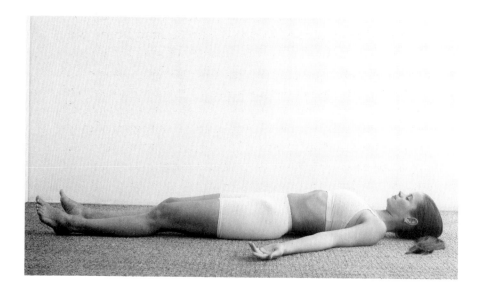

Afterword: A Time of Self-Renewal

AFTER READING THROUGH THIS BOOK, YOU'VE NO DOUBT COME TO understand that menstruation is more than the sum of its problems. Having your period every month does not automatically mean you have to have bad cramps or raging PMS, acne outbreaks or a bloated belly. With a little tender loving care each month, which includes a daily yoga practice and good eating habits, you can learn to celebrate your cycle instead of dreading it. Remember, menstruation embodies the essence of who you are as a woman and plays a major role in helping you discover the connection between your body and your emotions, between you and the world around you. It's time to stop thinking of your menstrual cycle as something that happens to you. Treat it as an ally, as a means of gauging how you've lived all month long, and as a natural monthly cleansing.

Above all, be observant. If you never take the time to listen to what your body needs, how can you know what causes your cramps? If you don't keep a monthly account of what you eat (or what's eating you emotionally), how will you know what brings on your premenstrual anxiety attack? Once you begin to see patterns—for instance, if you eat chocolate or drink coffee when you have PMS, you almost always get bad cramps; when you get a massage once a month, you don't feel as irritable just before your period—you'll have an easier time managing the discomfort and celebrating the benefits.

If you practice yoga daily or even several times a week, you'll discover that it helps you focus exclusively on yourself in a gentle, loving way. It may not stop your cramps from recurring or shrink your fibroids overnight, but it will transform the way you relate to those challenges. Your practice will nurture you and support you all month as it strengthens and nourishes your endocrine system. And just as important, it will teach you to heed the wisdom of your heart and the healing power of your mind. Namaste.

Resources

I HAVE INCLUDED BOOKS, MAGAZINES, VIDEOS, INFORMATION SOURCES, and everything else I could think of in this list of resources that might help you on your journey toward wellness and honoring your monthly cycle.

READING MATERIAL

This section includes the articles and publications mentioned in the book, as well as some others I think you may find useful.

Books

Borysenko, Joan. *A Woman's Book of Life: The Biology, Psychology, and Spirituality of the Feminine Life Cycle.* New York: Riverhead Books, 1996.

Crawford, Amanda McQuade. *Herbal Remedies for Women: Discovering Nature's Wonderful Secrets Just for Women.* Freedom, Calif.: Crossing Press, 1996.

Gladstar, Rosemary. *Herbal Healing for Women: Simple Home Remedies for Women of All Ages.* New York: Simon & Schuster, 1993.

Iyengar, B. K. S. *Light on Yoga: Yoga Dipika.* New York: Schocken Books, 1979.

———, trans. *Seventy Glorious Years of Yogacharya.* Puna, India: Light on Yoga Trust, 1990.

Iyengar, Geeta. *Yoga: A Gem for Women*. Palo Alto, Calif.: Timeless Books, 1990.

Lark, Susan. *Dr. Lark's Premenstrual Syndrome Self-Help Book: A Woman's Guide to Feeling Good All Month*. Berkeley, Calif.: Celestial Arts, 1993.

———. *Fibroid Tumor and Endometriosis Self-Help Book*. Berkeley, Calif.: Celestial Arts, 1995.

———. *Menstrual Cramps Self-Help Book: Effective Solutions for Pain and Discomfort Due to Menstrual Cramps and PMS*. Berkeley, Calif.: Celestial Arts, 1995.

———. *The PMS Self Help Book: A Woman's Guide*. Berkeley, Calif.: Celestial Arts, 1984.

Lasater, Judith. *Relax and Renew: Restful Yoga for Stressful Times*. Berkeley, Calif.: Rodmell Press, 1995.

Lonsdorf, Nancy, Veronica Butler, and Melanie Brown. *A Woman's Best Medicine: Health, Happiness, and Long Life through Ayurveda*. New York: Putnam, 1993.

Monro, Robin, R. Nagarathna, and H. R. Nagendra. *Yoga for Common Ailments*. New York: Simon & Schuster, 1990.

Northrup, Christiane. *Women's Bodies, Women's Wisdom: Creating Physical and Emotional Health and Healing*. New York: Bantam Books, 1998.

Pipher, Mary. *Reviving Ophelia: Saving the Selves of Adolescent Girls*. New York: Putnam, 1994.

Raman, Krishna. *A Matter of Health*. Madras, India: East-West Books, 1998. (Available through Iyengar yoga centers.)

Skilling, Johanna, and Eileen Hoffmann. *Fibroids: The Complete Guide to Taking Charge of Your Physical, Emotional, and Sexual Well-Being*. New York: Marlowe & Company, 2000.

Tiwari, Maya. *Ayurveda: A Life of Balance: The Complete Guide to Ayurvedic Nutrition and Body Types with Recipes*. Rochester, Vt.: Healing Arts Press, 1995.

Warshowsky, Allan, and Elena Oumano. *Healing Fibroids: A Doctor's Guide to a Natural Cure*. New York: Fireside Press, 2002.

Woodman, Marion, with Jill Mellick. *Coming Home to Myself: Daily Reflections for a Woman's Body and Soul*. Berkeley, Calif.: Conari Press, 1998.

Subscription Information for Journals, Magazines, and Newsletters

HerbalGram, P.O. Box 144345, Austin, TX 78714. Phone: (512) 926-4900; Web site: herbalgram.org.

The Herb Quarterly, 1041 Shary Circle, Concord, CA 94518. Web site: herbquarterly.com.

The Lark Letter, P.O. Box 60046, Potomac, MD 20897.

Yoga International. Phone: (800) 253-6243; Web site: himalayaninstitute.org.

Yoga Journal, 2054 University Ave., Berkeley, CA 94704. Phone: (800) 600-9642; Web site: yogajournal.com.

ASSOCIATIONS AND WEB SITES

The following organizations provide more detailed information on a variety of health issues and conditions.

American Botanical Council (ABC), P.O. Box 201660, Austin, TX 78720. Phone: (512) 926-4900; Web site: herbalgram.org.

Center for Uterine Fibroids, Brigham and Women's Hospital, Departments of Obstetrics/Gynecology and Pathology, 623 Thorn Building, 20 Shattuck St., Boston, MA 02115. Phone: (800) 722-5520 (ext. 80081); Web site: fibroids.net.

Endometriosis Association, 8585 N. 76th Pl., Milwaukee, WI 53223. Phone: (414) 355-2200; fax: (414) 355-6065; Web site: endometriosisassn. org and endometriosis.org.

Endometriosis Research Center, 630 Ibis Dr., Delray Beach, FL 33444. Phone: (561) 274-7442 or (800) 239-7280; fax: (561) 274-0931; Web site: www.endocenter.org; E-mail: EndoFL@aol.com.

Herb Research Foundation, 1007 Pearl St., #200, Boulder, CO 80302. Phone: (303) 449-2265; Web site: herbs.org.

National Black Woman's Health Project, 1211 Connecticut Ave. NW, #310, Washington, DC 20036. Phone: (202) 835-0117; Web site: www.blackwomenshealth.org.

National Institute of Mental Health, NIMH Public Inquiries, 6001 Executive Blvd., Rm. 8184, MSC 9663, Bethesda, MD 20892-9663. Phone: (301) 443-4513; Web site: www.nimh.nih.gov; E-mail: nimhinfo@nih.gov.

The Raj, Ayurveda Health Center, 1734 Jasmine Ave., Fairfield, IA 52556. Phone: (800) 248-9050, (641) 472-9580 in Iowa; E-mail: theraj@lisco.com.

Women's Health Research at the NICHD (National Institute of Child Health and Human Development), P.O. Box 3006, Rockville, MD 20847. Phone: (800) 370-2943; fax: (301) 496-7101; Web site: www.nichd.nih.gov; E-mail: NICHDInformationResourceCenter@mail.nih.gov.

Women's International Pharmacy, 5708 Monona Dr., Madison, WI 54716. Phone: (800) 279-5708; Web site: womensinternational.com; E-mail: info@womensinternational.com.

VIDEOS, AUDIOTAPES, AND OTHER PRODUCTS

Videos

AM and PM Yoga for Beginners with Rodney Yee and Patricia Walden (two-volume set)

Endometriosis: The Inside Story, produced by Belle Browne, R.N., is an Australian video. Available in the United States through endometriosis.org.

Flowing Yoga Postures for Beginners with Lilias Folan

Yoga for Round Bodies (volumes 1 and 2) with Linda DeMarco and Genia Pauli Haddon

Yoga Journal's Practice Series:

Yoga Practice: Introduction with Patricia Walden
Yoga Practice for Beginners with Patricia Walden
Yoga Practice for Flexibility with Patricia Walden
Yoga Practice for Strength with Rodney Yee
Yoga Practice for Relaxation with Patricia Walden and Rodney Yee
Yoga Practice for Energy with Rodney Yee
Yoga Practice for Meditation with Rodney Yee

Audiotapes

Discover Yoga with Lilias Folan
Discover Serenity with Lilias Folan

Products

The following mail-order companies offer a variety of items that may help you with your yoga practice, including yoga mats, blankets, blocks, bolsters, straps, inversion aids, and even clothing. Contact companies directly to find out what they carry.

Body Lift. Phone: (888) 243-3279; Web site: ageeasy.com.

Hugger Mugger Yoga Products. Phone: (800) 473-4888;
    Web site: www.huggermugger.com.

Lilias products. Web site: naturaljourneys.com.

Living Arts catalog. Phone: (800) 254-8464; Web site: www.gaiam.com.

Tools for Yoga. Phone: (888) 678-9642; Web site: toolsforyoga.com.

Yoga Accessories. Phone: (800) 990-9642; Web site: yogaaccessories.com.

Yoga Mats. Phone: (800) 720-9642; Web site: yogamats.com.

YogaPro. Phone: (800) 488-6414; Web site: yogapro.com.

Yoga Props. Phone: (888) 856-9642; Web site: yogaprops.net.

Yoga Shop 4U. Phone: (401) 353-3513; Web site: yogashop4u.com.

Yoga Wear. Phone: (800) 217-0006; Web site: mariewright.net.

Acknowledgments

WRITING THIS BOOK REMINDS ME THAT TEAMWORK IS ALWAYS preferable to a solitary effort. I'm blessed to have the best team ever! First and foremost, of course, is Patricia Walden, my teacher, my writing partner, and most important, my friend. An internationally recognized expert in women's health, Patricia not only provided the sequences in this book, but shared her research and the hands-on experience she's had with hundreds of yoga students of all ages. I have a deep sense of gratitude for the work of B. K. S. Iyengar, a modern-day yogi and therapeutic genius, and his daughter Geeta, a pioneer in the field of women's health and yoga. Patricia's inspiration and teachings come from her close association with the Iyengars; without their groundbreaking work, this book (like so many others) would simply not have been possible.

Then we have the publishing cast of experts who believed in this project from the very beginning: my agent, Joe Spieler, along with Peter Turner and Jonathan Green at Shambhala Publications, who took care of all the details. My copyeditors, Jim Keough and Karen Steib, always make me sound much better than I should. Illustrator Jennifer Devine's drawings grace these pages and illuminate the text. Ben Gleason kept track of details and helped keep the book on schedule. Designers Steve Dyer and Greta Sibley created a beautiful product, and Peter Bermudes's and Julie Saidenberg's unbridled enthusiasm as a publicist ensures that the whole world embraces it. And thanks, of course, to Emily Bower, my editor, who always makes me feel that anything's possible. She's the best.

Yoga photographer David Martinez was also an integral part of this project. I thank him from the bottom of my heart for his patience and unflappability and his choice of assistants—Aneata Ferguson and Charlie Nucci. I am so grateful to Amy Stone and Winnie Chen. Both of these lovely yoginis put their own lives and teaching schedules on hold to model the poses you see in these pages. Brenda Beebe, owner of Yoga Mats in San Francisco, is also a good friend who generously provided all the props featured in the sequences.

I have learned so much from the works of other women, particularly Christiane Northrup, M.D.; Susan Lark, M.D.; and Nancy Lonsdorf, M.D.; I am pleased to be able to honor them and their research in these pages. I am indebted to Alice Damar, Ph.D., of Harvard University for agreeing to write the foreword—I'm a longtime admirer of her work. I'm also thankful to all the teachers who work with me at the San Francisco Bay Club and Bay Club Marin and listened to me carry on about menstruation month after month—especially Lee Monozon; Leigh Threlkel; Dina Amsterdam; Amy Stone; and my lovely assistant, Erin Peary, who kept things running while I was hiding out at my computer. Thanks also to Nestor Fernandez and Jim Gerber (my "bosses"), who gave me time off to write, and to my writing buddies—Stephen Cope, Kathryn Arnold, Jennifer Barrett, and Anne Cushman—who believed in me no matter what. Above all, I want to honor my teachers who have contributed more than they know to my own understanding of this deep and abiding practice. They have singly and collectively held me in their hearts and contributed greatly to my own healing: Patricia Sullivan, Sarah Powers, Sharon Gannon, Bri. Maya Tiwari, Marion Woodman, Ty Powers, Sharon Salzburg, Patty Craves, and Janice Gates.

Finally, I would never have completed this book without the love and support I get at home, especially from my husband and on-site editor, Jim Keough. Although our daughters, Sarah and Megan, are no longer living nearby, their cheerleading from across the miles kept me going, and their invitations to visit provided the right amount of distraction.

It's entirely possible that I've inadvertently left someone out. If so, please know it was an unintentional omission and your name will no doubt surface in my brain and warm my heart the minute this book goes to press!

Index